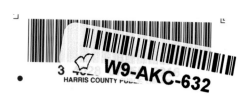

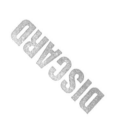

THE TRUTH ABOUT ALCOHOL

SECOND EDITION

Robert N. Golden, M.D.
University of Wisconsin–Madison
General Editor

Fred L. Peterson, Ph.D.
University of Texas–Austin
General Editor

Barry Youngerman
Principal Author

Heath Dingwell
Contributing Author

William Kane, Ph.D.
University of New Mexico
Adviser to the First Edition

Mark J. Kittleson, Ph.D.
Southern Illinois University
Adviser to the First Edition

Richelle Rennegarbe, Ph.D.
McKendree College
Adviser

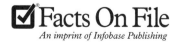

Facts On File
An imprint of Infobase Publishing

The Truth About Alcohol, Second Edition

Facts On File, Inc.
An imprint of Infobase Publishing
132 West 31st Street
New York NY 10001

Library of Congress Cataloging-in-Publication Data

Youngerman, Barry.
    The truth about alcohol / Barry Youngerman, principal author ; Heath Dingwell, contributing author ; Robert N. Golden, general editor, Fred Peterson, general editor ; Richelle Rennegarbe, advisor. − 2nd ed.
        p. cm.
    Rev. ed. of: Truth about alcohol / Mark J. Kittleson, general editor. c2005.
    Includes bibliographical references and index.
    ISBN-13: 978-0-8160-7639-0 (hardcover : alk. paper)
    ISBN-10: 0-8160-7639-1 (hardcover : alk. paper) 1. Teenagers−Alcohol use. 2. Alcoholism−Prevention. I. Dingwell, Heath. II. Golden, Robert N. III. Peterson, Fred. IV. Truth about alcohol. V. Title.
    RJ506.D78T78 2010
    362.292'0835−dc22
                                                        2009053476

Facts On File books are available at special discounts when purchased in bulk quantities for businesses, associations, institutions, or sales promotions. Please call our Special Sales Department in New York at (212) 967-8800 or (800) 322-8755.

You can find Facts On File on the World Wide Web at http://www.factsonfile.com

Text design by David Strelecky
Composition by Mary Susan Ryan-Flynn
Cover printed by Art Print, Taylor, Pa.
Book printed and bound by Maple Press, York, Pa.
Date printed: September 2010
Printed in the United States of America

10 9 8 7 6 5 4 3 2 1

This book is printed on acid-free paper.

CONTENTS

LIST OF ILLUSTRATIONS

PREFACE

THE TRUTH ABOUT series—updated and expanded to include 20 volumes—seeks to identify the most pressing health issues and social challenges confronting our nation's youth. Adolescence is the period between the onset of puberty and the attainment of adult roles and responsibilities. Adolescence is also a time of storm, stress, and risk taking for many young people. During adolescence, a person's health is influenced by biological, psychological, and social factors, all of which interact with one's environment—family, peers, school, and community. It is a time when teenagers experience profound changes.

With the latest available statistics and new insights that have emerged from ongoing research, the Truth About series seeks to help young people build a foundation of information as they face some of the challenges that will affect their health and well-being. These challenges include high-risk behaviors, such as alcohol, tobacco, and other drug use; sexual behaviors that can lead to adolescent pregnancy and sexually transmitted diseases (STDs), such as HIV/AIDS; mental health concerns, such as depression and suicide; learning disorders and disabilities, which are often associated with school failures and school drop-outs; serious family problems, including domestic violence and abuse; and lifestyle factors, which increase adolescents' risk for noncommunicable diseases, such as diabetes and cardiovascular disease, among others.

Broader underlying factors also influence adolescent health. These include socioeconomic circumstances, such as poverty, available health care, and the political and social situations in which young people live. Although these factors can negatively affect adolescent health and well-being, as well as school performance, many of these negative health outcomes are preventable with the proper knowledge and information.

With prevention in mind, the writers and editors of each topical volume in the Truth About series have tried to provide cutting-edge information that is supported by research and scientific evidence. Vital facts are presented that inform youth about the challenges experienced during adolescence, while special features seek to dispel common myths and misconceptions. Some of the main topics explored include abuse, alcohol, death and dying, divorce, drugs, eating disorders, family life, fear and depression, rape, sexual behavior and unplanned pregnancy, smoking, and violence. All volumes discuss risk-taking behaviors and their consequences, healthy choices, prevention, available treatments, and where to get help.

In this new edition of the series, we also have added eight new titles in areas of increasing significance to today's youth. ADHD, or attention-deficit/hyperactivity disorder, and learning disorders are diagnosed with increasing frequency, and many students have observed or know of classmates receiving treatment for these conditions, even if they have not themselves received this diagnosis. Gambling is gaining currency in our culture, as casinos open and expand in many parts of the country, and the Internet offers easy access for this addictive behavior. Another consequence of our increasingly "online" society, unfortunately, is the presence of online predators. Environmental hazards represent yet another danger, and it is important to provide unbiased information about this topic to our youth. Suicide, which for many years has been a "silent epidemic," is now gaining recognition as a major public health problem throughout the life span, including the teenage and young-adult years. We now also offer an overview of illness and disease in a volume that includes the major conditions of particular interest and concern to youth. In addition to illness, however, it is essential to emphasize health and its promotion, and this is especially apparent in the volumes on physical fitness and stress management.

It is our intent that each book serve as an accessible, authoritative resource to which young people can turn for accurate and meaningful answers to their specific questions. The series can help them research particular problems and provide an up-to-date evidence base. It is also designed with parents, teachers, and counselors in mind, so that they have a reliable resource that they can share with youth who seek their guidance.

Finally, we have tried to provide unbiased facts rather than subjective opinions. Our goal is to help elevate the health of the public with an emphasis on its most precious component—its youth. As young people face the challenges of an increasingly complex world, we as educators want them to be armed with the most powerful weapon available—knowledge.

Robert N. Golden, M.D.
Fred L. Peterson, Ph.D.
General Editors

HOW TO USE THIS BOOK

NOTE TO STUDENTS

Knowledge is power. By possessing knowledge you have the ability to make decisions, ask follow-up questions, or know where to go to obtain more information. In the world of health that is power! That is the purpose of this book—to provide you the power you need to obtain unbiased, accurate information and *The Truth About Alcohol.*

Topics in each volume of The Truth About are arranged in alphabetical order, from *A* to *Z*. Each of these entries defines its topic and explains in detail the particular issue. At the end of most entries are cross-references to related topics. A list of all topics by letter can be found in the table of contents or at the back of the book in the index.

How have these books been compiled? First, the publisher worked with me to identify some of the country's leading authorities on key issues in health education. These individuals were asked to identify some of the major concerns that young people have about such topics. The writers read the literature, spoke with health experts, and incorporated their own life and professional experiences to pull together the most up-to-date information on health issues, particularly those of interest to adolescents and of concern in Healthy People 2010.

Throughout the alphabetical entries, the reader will find sidebars that separate fact from fiction. There are question-and-answer boxes that attempt to address the most common questions that youth ask about sensitive topics. In addition, readers will find a special feature called "Teens Speak"—case studies of teens with personal stories related to the topic in hand.

This may be one of the most important books you will ever read. Please share it with your friends, families, teachers, and classmates. Remember, you possess the power to control your future. One way to affect your course is through the acquisition of knowledge. Good luck and keep healthy.

NOTE TO LIBRARIANS

This book, along with the rest of the series, The Truth About, serves as a wonderful resource for young researchers. It contains a variety of facts, case studies, and further readings that the reader can use to help answer questions, formulate new questions, or determine where to go to find more information. Even though the topics may be considered delicate by some, do not be afraid to ask patrons if they have questions. Feel free to direct them to the appropriate sources, but do not press them if you encounter reluctance. The best we can do as educators is to let young people know that we are there when they need us.

Mark J. Kittleson, Ph.D.
General Editor of the First Edition

ADDICTIVE BEHAVIORS AND ALCOHOL

In common speech, the term *heavy drinking* can be very vague. However, according to the National Institute of Alcohol Abuse and Alcoholism, a heavy drinker consumes five or more drinks (or sometimes four, for a woman) on at least five different occasions during a month. In other words, anyone who drinks a six-pack of beer once or twice every weekend is considered a heavy drinker.

Some adults can be heavy drinkers for years without falling into the category of alcohol abusers, people who consume alcohol excessively. They may always drink in a pleasant social setting, never drive after drinking, and be responsible spouses, parents, and employees. For young people, however, heavy drinking is usually very difficult to manage and is generally associated with abuse.

NEW IN THE REVISED EDITION

Alcohol abuse is still a serious social problem. In this new edition of *The Truth About Alcohol,* you will find updated statistics and new entries to help you recognize the behaviors that lead to heavy drinking.

Underage drinking continues to be prevalent, although there is some good news to report. In 1992, 51.3 percent of 12th-grade students admitted to drinking alcohol within the past month. By 2007, however, this number had decreased to 44.4 percent. The number of students who admitted to being drunk decreased from 29.9 in 1992 to 28.7 percent in 2007. It appears, however, that while overall drinking among 12th-graders is down, those who do drink often get drunk.

One of the reasons that drinking is widespread is that the alcohol industry is estimated to spend $2 billion a year on advertising in the media, with figures rising to $6 billion a year when every form of advertising is taken into account. Progress, however, has been made to prevent exposing youth to commercials for alcohol. At present, only approximately 6 percent of advertising for alcohol on television shows is directed primarily at youth.

Problems abound because of alcohol use and abuse. It plays a role in homicides, suicides, domestic violence, cancer, and deaths due to automobile and other accidents. In fact, tens of thousands of people die every year due to alcohol-related causes and even more are injured.

To help examine some of the newest information on the problems stemming from alcohol use, there are seven new entries in this edition. The first focuses on the relationship between alcohol and depression, which is complicated. Alcohol use certainly influences a person's level of depression. At the same time, depression increases the odds of alcohol use and abuse.

Alcohol poisoning is another new entry. Many people do not realize that alcohol is a poison to the body. It is a foreign substance that the body has to break down and eliminate. Alcohol poisoning occurs when someone drinks so much alcohol in a short period of time that the body cannot handle it. When this happens, a person can die if not treated properly.

The subject of alcohol tolerance has also been added to this edition. People who drink regularly usually build a tolerance to alcohol. This means it takes more alcohol to produce the hypnotic, or sedative, effects from drinking. There are several factors contributing to tolerance. Gender, body mass, frequency of drinking, and the amount one drinks all influence alcohol tolerance.

Alcohol withdrawal is another new addition to this book. A **chronic** drinker forces his or her body to try to work properly when alcohol is present. Because alcohol is a **depressant,** various organs and systems within the body need to work harder. Alcohol withdrawal occurs when a chronic drinker stops drinking. Withdrawing from alcohol is a quicker process for the body than adapting to the constant presence of alcohol. This process can be violent as the body starts readjusting to the lack of alcohol. In a sense, the body is thrown into a state of shock. If withdrawal from alcohol is not treated properly, it can potentially kill a person.

Another new entry focuses on racial and ethnic differences associated with alcohol use. Alcohol use, abuse, and treatment differ across racial and ethnic groups. Generally speaking, whites are more likely to use and abuse alcohol than Hispanics, blacks, Asians, and other groups. At the same time, they are also in a better position to receive alcohol counseling when necessary.

Another new topic focuses on codependency, an unhealthy relationship between someone with an alcohol problem and that person's partner (e.g., girlfriend, boyfriend, fiancé[e], spouse). Codependents were once typically viewed as being women, although it is now acknowledged that men can also be codependent. Research indicates that self-esteem is one of the keys in understanding codependency. Those with low self-esteem are more likely to stay in bad relationships because they feel they cannot do better. However, other research indicates that behaviors traditionally viewed as "codependent" are better seen as coping mechanisms to help handle a troubled relationship.

Alcohol screening is the last new entry to this edition. Tools known as assessments are available to help determine if someone has a drinking problem. These tools are primarily designed for health-care professionals and can be used in a variety of settings. The most common assessments are discussed here. They include the ASSIST, AUDIT, MAST, and CAGE, all reliable measure aspects of problem drinking and alcoholism.

THE IMPACT OF ALCOHOL

The different impact that alcohol has on different individuals makes it difficult to generalize when discussing alcohol use, abuse, and **addiction:** What affects one person one way may affect someone else differently. Still, by definition, alcohol abuse is always a problem behavior. The National Institute of Alcohol Abuse and Alcoholism defines the term as "a pattern of drinking that results in one or more of the following situations within a 12-month period:

- Failure to fulfill major work, school, or home responsibilities;
- Drinking in situations that are physically dangerous, such as while driving a car or operating machinery;
- Having recurring alcohol-related legal problems, such as being arrested for driving under the influence of alcohol or for physically hurting someone while drunk; and
- Continued drinking despite having ongoing relationship problems that are caused or worsened by the drinking."

A person can abuse alcohol without being an **alcoholic,** that is, without the physical dependence. The cravings may not be overpowering, and the person may be able to stop drinking on any one occasion. However, the abusive behavior patterns are difficult to overcome, and it may be difficult for alcohol abusers to develop safe drinking behaviors.

DEFINITIONS OF DRINKING BEHAVIORS

The terms *alcohol addiction, alcohol dependency,* and *alcoholism* are often used to mean the same thing. However, they can be used to highlight different aspects of the same behavior.

The term *addiction* can be used for any drug, as well as for other patterns of behavior such as gambling. Addiction is a chronic disease in which a person has a physical and psychological need or craving for the substance or behavior. It lasts for a long period of time and is difficult or impossible to cure. It can be controlled, but relapses are common, in which the person slips back into his or her old, problematic behavior.

Binge drinking refers to a period of drinking five or more drinks at one sitting; this is sometimes called heavy episodic drinking—"episodic" because it only happens now and then. Some reports consider a woman to be engaged in binge drinking if she drinks *four* or more drinks at one time.

Dependency is a term used only for drug-related addictions. It usually refers to a physical condition in the addict's brain and other organs. Anyone who is dependent on a drug needs periodic doses of the drug just to avoid painful, uncomfortable, or frightening symptoms. Those symptoms are summed up in the term *withdrawal,* which is discussed later in this section.

Alcoholism means an addiction to alcohol. It includes a strong craving or compulsion to drink at regular intervals (every day, for many alcoholics, or just periodically, for example, on weekends, for others). It includes a loss of control; once an alcoholic takes one drink, he or she generally cannot stop. Alcoholics also have a physical dependence on the drug and experience withdrawal symptoms if they stop drinking.

Some alcoholics vary their behaviors between episodes of excessive drinking and periods of sobriety. Alcoholics who have overcome their cravings and have been sober for a long period of time are usually considered "alcoholics in recovery."

Tolerance

People who drink a large amount of alcohol, especially those who have become dependent on alcohol, usually develop a degree of **tolerance**. People who need to drink more to get the same mental effect, or who get less of a buzz when they drink their usual amount, probably have an acquired tolerance to alcohol. They say things like, "I really can hold my liquor," or "I can drink you under the table."

Tolerance occurs as the brain and nervous system become accustomed to alcohol. The nerve cells adapt their normal functioning to compensate for the effects of the drug. However, even in the brain, the tolerance can only go so far. A heavy drinker may need more alcohol to get drunk but only a little bit more to black out, go into a coma, or die. Also, as tolerance develops and drinkers continually increase their dose, the brain may adjust but other organs can be seriously damaged.

An alcoholic's liver can develop **metabolic tolerance** to alcohol by learning to break down or metabolize a larger amount of the substance in a given period of time than the liver of a nonalcoholic. However, none of the other vital organs are so flexible. A given amount of alcohol inflicts the same amount of damage to an alcoholic's stomach, heart, arteries, bone, and other organs as it does with a casual drinker, even if the alcoholic never feels drunk.

A high degree of tolerance can give heavy drinkers a false sense of security. They may not feel drunk, but in all likelihood their coordination, reflexes, and judgment are impaired. People who develop a high tolerance to alcohol should not be fooled into thinking that they can safely drive or perform other difficult or dangerous tasks just because they don't feel drunk.

Tolerance may vary with the environment. Some people can drive home along a familiar route even after a couple of drinks. But if they try a different route, the same level of blood alcohol can cause much greater impairment.

Alcoholics often lose their high level of tolerance after an extended period of time, and then even one drink makes them drunk. This may be a sign of liver damage and should not be ignored. It also can lead to severe, unexpected intoxication, which is especially dangerous when driving.

Withdrawal

When alcoholics or heavy drinkers suddenly stop drinking, or when they drastically cut back on the amount they drink, they usually experience some form of withdrawal. *Withdrawal* refers to the combination of painful and uncomfortable symptoms they feel as their bodies try to re-adapt to an alcohol-free bloodstream.

When the brain and nervous system are suddenly deprived of alcohol, they quickly try to readjust to their normal, drug-free behavior. This sounds simple, but it is very unpleasant to experience. According to scientists, the nerve cells in the brain become accustomed to working extra hard to overcome the depressing effects of alcohol. For a while, they continue to work overtime, but without alcohol to slow them down, they are in a super-excited state.

A few hours after the last drink, the patient may feel weak, shaky, and anxious, and usually suffers from headache, nausea, and stomach cramps. Somewhat later, he or she begins to feel agitated and starts to crave another drink. As the hours go by, severe **tremors,** or shaking, may develop, followed by **hallucinations**—seeing and hearing things that aren't there.

In more severe cases, brain seizures may occur, and need to be treated immediately with powerful drugs. The worst-case scenario is called **delirium tremens,** or the D.T.'s. These intense, terrifying hallucinations continue for three to four days, accompanied by high fevers and extremely aggressive behavior. A century ago, up to 40 percent of D.T. cases resulted in death; improvements in treatment have reduced the rate to 5 percent, according to a 1998 study reported in the *Southern Medical Journal.*

The majority of cases of severe withdrawal occur in older people who have been drinking for years. But people as young as 20 also can experience withdrawal, depending on how much and how long they have been drinking.

Teens should also bear in mind that even a mild withdrawal could set the stage for more severe problems later on, due to the **kindling effect,** which means that when alcoholics go through withdrawal more than once, the symptoms often get more severe each time. The nerve cells seem to become kindled—they are not charged up enough to cause problems now but any additional charge in the future could push them over the top. Evidence suggests that people who show this effect are in greater danger of relapse (returning to alcohol abuse) and also are more likely to suffer brain damage.

Even relatively mild cases of withdrawal may need medical attention. Anyone who makes the courageous decision to fight alcohol dependency should arrange to have help in advance.

WHAT ARE THE SYMPTOMS AND BEHAVIORS OF ALCOHOL ABUSE AND ALCOHOLISM?

Teenagers are among alcohol's most obvious victims. When young people drink, lots of bad things often happen—to the drinkers and to those around them. As a result, Congress and state legislators have made it illegal to sell or serve alcohol in the United States to people under 21 years old. However, the laws have not been easy to enforce, and underage drinking continues.

In fact, many kids have fallen into dangerous habits of heavy drinking, abuse, and even addiction. Other kids are at risk of doing the same; many of them may not even be aware of the dangers they face.

In the 22 articles that follow on the problems associated with alcohol and addiction, you can read about the main types of harmful alcohol-related behavior and learn how common they are among young people. You also can discover information on the risk factors for alcohol abuse, and the signs that show whether you or someone you know has begun to develop addictive problems with alcohol. This information may help keep you out of harm's way, or help you start dealing with any problems you may already have.

The signs of alcohol abuse

Some alcoholics are so skilled at concealing their problem that even friends, family members, or coworkers may not suspect the extent of their drinking. In the majority of cases, however, especially with younger drinkers, some signs of alcohol abuse can be a tip-off to concerned loved ones. Here are some of them:

- Drinking alone
- Being unable to cut back
- Drinking in the morning
- Keeping a supply of alcohol in a hidden place
- Wishing they had a drink
- Going to school or work drunk
- Drinking even while taking prescription drugs, against the doctor's orders
- Gulping instead of sipping alcohol
- Lying to family and friends about drinking
- Finding excuses to drink
- Drinking more than they intended
- Saying it's just a phase
- Drinking to escape problems, or to fall asleep
- Having blackouts
- Spending large amounts of time sleeping off hangovers
- Losing interest in schoolwork and starting to fall behind
- Avoiding friends who don't drink
- Feeling tired all the time without being ill
- Feeling more irritable than usual
- Getting angry if someone raises the subject of your drinking

The stages of drinking problems

Every human being possesses his or her own physical, psychological, and social makeup. Among people who drink alcohol, not everyone develops exactly the same habits. Still, many people who become alcoholics do seem to follow a particular pattern. This is known as **progression**, or moving from one stage to another, more serious stage.

There are different definitions of the stages. The National Council on Alcoholism and Drug Dependence states, "The typical progression from alcohol use to addiction involves the following stages:

- Experimental stage: curiosity about the effects of alcohol causes the user to try alcohol one or more times;

- Social stage: alcohol is used occasionally in social situations such as parties or with friends;

- Dependent stage: the user becomes obsessed with alcohol and consumes it regularly, often alone; and

- Chronic stage: the user feels constant emotional or physical pain, which can be lessened only by alcohol."

ADDICTING SUBSTANCES AMONG TEENS: WHERE DOES ALCOHOL RANK?

Despite all the attention that marijuana, cocaine, club drugs, and other illegal substances get in the media, alcohol remains the most widely used—and abused—addicting drug among young Americans, even including tobacco. The 2007 Monitoring the Future Survey of the National Institute on Drug Abuse found that nearly twice as many eighth, 10th, and 12th graders had consumed alcohol in the previous month than had smoked cigarettes (15.9, 33.4, and 44.4 percent compared with 7.1, 14.0, and 21.6 percent).

Experts may debate whether one particular drug is more or less addictive than another; that is, whether a user would find it harder to give up alcohol or, for example, marijuana. That fact is hard to determine, but the number of teenagers who suffer from alcohol abuse dwarfs the numbers for any other drug—showing that alcohol use is a serious problem.

The latest figures, according to the National Household Survey on Drug Abuse (NHSDA), a project of the federal Department of Health and Human Services that gets its information from families themselves, reported that in 2007, 6.9 percent of all young people aged 12–17 were heavy drinkers. According to the NHSDA, a heavy drinker had "five or more drinks on the same occasion at least five different days in the past

30 days." In addition, another 22.3 percent were binge drinkers, who had five or more drinks on the same occasion in that same 30-day period.

This adds up to a large number of young people—more than 5 million teenage alcohol abusers, according to the National Institute on Alcohol Abuse and Alcoholism (NIAAA). Of course, not all of these individuals are addicted. With luck, most of the bingers will avoid becoming addicted. In 2003–04, according to the Substance Abuse and Mental Health Services Administration (SAMHSA), 111,000 adolescents under age 17 alcohol received treatment for alcohol abuse in the United States.

Compare those facts to other drugs. Each year, Monitoring the Future, a project under the U.S. Department of Health and Human Services, surveys about 50,000 kids in grades 8, 10, and 12 about their use of drugs, including alcohol and tobacco. The good news is that nearly every drug, including alcohol, saw small but significant declines in use in the past few years. But the pattern remains the same—alcohol is abused more than any other drug. In fact, alcohol is abused more than all illicit drugs combined, including marijuana, cocaine, inhalants, hallucinogens (such as LSD), ecstasy, heroin, **amphetamines**, barbiturates, and tranquilizers.

In 2007, Monitoring the Future found that, among 12th graders, 44.4 percent had used alcohol at least once and 28.7 percent had gotten drunk in the previous 30 days, as compared with 21.9 percent who used *any illicit drugs*. Over the course of the year, 66.4 percent had used alcohol, 46.1 percent had gotten drunk, and 35.9 percent had used any illicit drugs.

WHAT ARE THE RISK FACTORS?

A number of **risk factors**, or causes, may influence a teen who has experimented with alcohol to lose control and become dependent. Some of these causes, such as family history and friends' behavior, are beyond the person's control. However, there is always *something* a person can do to limit the impact of these factors and prevent them from running his or her life.

Family history

Perhaps the greatest single risk factor for alcohol abuse is a family history of alcoholism. People have long noticed that alcohol abuse runs in families, but they didn't know how it was passed along from one generation to the next. Was it a behavior pattern that children learned from watching their parents, or was it some inherited chemical factor that made certain people more susceptible to the dangers of alcohol? Or was it some combination of both factors?

By now, the majority of scientists who have studied the subject believe that the family's genes are responsible for alcoholism in families.

Studies of identical twins have found that if one twin is alcoholic, the other is quite likely to be alcoholic too. Other studies have found that kids from alcoholic families tend to have alcohol problems even if adopted and raised by nonalcoholics—and vice-versa.

Take note that the *majority* of children from families with a history of alcoholism do *not* themselves become alcoholic. However, more of them do than children of nonalcoholic families. According to alcohol researcher D. W. Goodwin, 20 to 25 percent of sons and brothers of alcoholics, and 5 percent of daughters and sisters of alcoholics, become alcoholics themselves. Also, these kids tend to become alcohol abusers and alcoholics at an earlier age than other people, and may suffer a more severe form of the disease.

Friends who drink

Most people are influenced by their friends, for better or worse. Unfortunately, this goes for alcohol abuse as well. If your circle of friends drinks, you may find it difficult to resist. Even if you don't become dependent, drinking among groups of teenagers often takes abusive forms.

You may believe you are strong enough to resist the influence of your friends. However, if you feel you are at risk for alcohol problems, due to family background or other factors, you may want to make a point of staying away from a circle of friends who drink.

Home and school

Problems at home and at school can sometimes lead to alcohol abuse. Most people do not try to escape their problems with drugs, but some do take that path. Alcohol, like many other drugs, may seem to help "get your mind off" your troubles. If your family is going through a rough period, such as an impending divorce; if your schoolwork has not been up to potential lately; or if you have broken up with a boyfriend or girlfriend, you may be tempted to escape your worries about these problems. This behavior can put you at risk for substance abuse.

The real danger is that you may come to think that alcohol is the only way to relieve your feelings of sadness or anxiety. If you feel that way, you are at very high risk of becoming dependent.

At times like these, becoming aware of your behaviors is even more important. Try to find healthy alternatives, such as sports or community service, to give yourself a little perspective. Always bear in mind that whatever your other problems may be, they will not be helped by adding alcohol to the situation.

Psychological factors

Adolescents with emotional problems are also at greater risk for alcohol abuse—just as troubled adults are. People who suffer from long-term depression are considered to be at risk; so are people who have difficulty coping with the normal problems and challenges of teen life.

For example, teens who feel insecure about their looks or social skills may turn to alcohol in the belief that getting drunk will help them overcome their shyness or inhibition. Other kids, who feel too much pressure to achieve, for example from parents, teachers, or coaches, might try to relieve the pressure by turning to alcohol.

Not every teenage alcoholic started out as an emotionally troubled child. Some drink as a way to feel independent or to stand up to authority. Although most people will not progress from the rebellious stage to alcoholism, if someone is at risk due to other factors, she or he should probably try to find more appropriate ways of acting grown up. Some teenagers say frankly that they drink because they choose to get drunk. You can't fault their honesty, but you can ask them a simple question: If they get drunk on a regular basis, are they really in control of their behavior?

Age of onset

Researchers have found that the younger a child is when he or she begins to drink, the more likely he or she is to become dependent on alcohol. Very few of these young kids expect to become addicted.

Not all kids who take their first drink at a very early age become dependent on alcohol, but there does seem to be a pattern, as indicated in two different surveys done at a 10-year interval. A 1991 report by the American Academy of Pediatrics found that one out of seven fourth graders (who are mostly nine years old) had already become drunk at least once. Ten years later, the National Household Survey found that one out of seven of the same age cohort, who were now 19 years old, were heavy drinkers. According to the National Survey of Drug Use and Health, in 2007, approximately 21.5 percent of this age cohort were heavy drinkers. That is slightly more than one in five people, indicating more of this group—now 24 to 25 years old—had become heavy drinkers since 2001.

Given their smaller size, children absorb alcohol into their bloodstream at a faster rate than older kids or adults. They become drunk sooner and remain drunk for a longer period of time. The toxic effects on the young nervous system, which is still developing, are likely to be more serious too. These drinkers may easily become physically tolerant, or addicted, to alcohol.

The circumstances of a child or teen's first alcohol experiences are also very important in determining how they behave in the future. In many foreign countries and among many immigrant communities in the United States, parents allow children, or even encourage them, to taste beer, wine, or even liquor at social or religious occasions. For years, researchers found lower levels of alcoholism among the children of first- or second-generation Americans with Italian, Greek, Chinese, and Jewish origins, who generally follow those traditions. Important family milestones were celebrated with a round of drinks and toasts.

For many Catholics and Jews, drinking wine plays an important role in religious ceremonies. For example, wine is usually served at the Passover seder in Jewish homes and at Christmas dinner among Italians, and kids are allowed to partake. For such kids, the researchers believe, alcohol is not a "forbidden fruit" associated with rebellion, but just another part of the traditional diet.

Experts can argue about whether such practices, if adopted in the future by all Americans, would reduce alcoholism. However, in today's world, very young drinkers usually have their first drink outside the home, which exposes them to a high level of risk.

REHABILITATION PROGRAMS

If these signs helped you realize that someone you know—perhaps yourself—has a problem with alcohol, do not despair. Although there is still much that doctors and treatment professionals do not know, many options are available to people who want to deal with their alcohol abuse.

They might first want to read the entries in this book on *Self-Help Programs* and *Recovery and Treatment*. Then they should turn to family and friends for guidance and moral support, if they feel they can. They also may need help from an organized treatment program. Many programs are available, so they may even need help in selecting which program in their area is best for them. For information on these options, please see *Hotlines and Help Sites* at the end of this book.

Teens who are fighting an addiction to alcohol may have special issues in trying to rebuild their lives. But they may have certain advantages too.

Compared to the family members of adult alcoholics, families of recovering teenagers may be more able and willing to forgive their teen for the destructive behavior of the past. After all, giving support is part of what it means to be a parent. However, many parents lose patience, and may eventually "wash their hands" of their alcoholic children, if the kids don't make a major effort to do their part in recovery.

Teachers and school staff are more likely to give the recovering alcoholic another chance, compared to employers, who may have suffered financial loss from an alcoholic employee. Finally, teenagers who have overcome alcohol addiction still have long lives ahead of them. True, no one can give them back the time they wasted, but with work and determination, they can look forward to experiencing the challenges of adult life with the wisdom and strength that recovery can sometimes give.

RISKY BUSINESS SELF-TEST

Most people in the early stages of alcohol dependence are blissfully unaware that they have a problem, or they may be trying hard not to admit it to themselves. If you drink more than once in a while, you might want to ask yourself the following 20 questions. On a piece of paper, keep a record of your answers—"yes" or "no."

Personality changes

Although other causes may account for these issues, alcohol might well be one.

- Am I losing interest in schoolwork and starting to fall behind?
- Do I avoid my old friends who don't drink?
- Do I feel tired all the time, without being ill?
- Do I feel more irritable than in the past?
- Do I get angry if someone asks me any of the questions above?
- Do I get angry if someone raises the subject of my drinking alcohol?
- Do I find myself lying to family and friends about how often and how much I drink?

Changes in drinking patterns

These are usually signs of alcohol abuse.

- Do I drink alone?
- Do I drink in the morning?
- Do I go to school or work drunk?
- Do I drink even while taking prescription drugs, against doctor's orders?

- Do I drink to escape problems, or to fall asleep?
- Do I explain my drinking as "just a phase"?
- Do I gulp instead of sip alcohol?
- Do I have blackouts, forgetting what happened while I was drinking?
- Do I spend a lot of time sleeping off hangovers?

Cravings and loss of control

These are signs that abuse may be turning into addiction:

- Do I wind up drinking more than I intended when I picked up the first glass?
- Do I keep a supply of alcohol in a hidden place?
- Do I find myself wishing I had a drink?
- Do I look for excuses to drink?

When counting up all of your answers, did you answer "yes" to more than 15 questions? If so, you should talk with someone about your drinking behaviors. (Remember, a drinking buddy is not a good choice here, unless he or she also is asking serious questions.) If *any* of the behaviors in the last two groups looks familiar to you, you should seek help.

If you still are not sure you or someone you care about has a problem, here's another question to ask yourself: Did any of the following sentences pop into your head as you read the list above? These are things that alcoholics in denial tend to say:

- I'll never become an alcoholic because when I drink too much, I get sick before I can get really bombed.
- Alcoholics look like sloppy drunks; I never look like that, so I can't be addicted.
- I only drink to please my friends; I can stop whenever I want to.
- Alcoholism doesn't run in my family.
- I never drink on school nights.
- I only drink on weekends.
- I only drink at parties.

All these statements may be true, yet you still may have an alcohol problem. If you have any doubts, talk about it with someone you trust.

A-TO-Z ENTRIES

■ ADVERTISING AND COUNTERADVERTISING CAMPAIGNS

Attempts to reach a target market by designing a series of advertisements and placing them in various media. As a typical teenager, you have seen many TV commercials promoting beer. You've seen good-looking, healthy young actors on the TV screen who seem to know how to enjoy life—and they are depicted drinking beer. They never feel lonely or awkward. They always are surrounded by happy, supportive friends.

How much do these ads influence you, or other teenagers? Experts disagree. Yet whether or not the ads influence *most* people, *you* can maintain your own independence if you remain critically aware of the "information" you receive about alcohol.

ARE TEENS TARGETED?

For years, critics have accused the makers of beer and other alcoholic beverages of deliberately promoting their products to the underage market. Are they right?

No one has actually proven that the industry is in fact trying to get kids to drink—or to drink more than they already do. Furthermore, there is no clear-cut evidence that the ads actually do influence drinking behavior.

Everyone agrees, however, that the average teenager is exposed to several hundred alcohol commercials every year. The Center on Alcohol Marketing and Youth, part of Georgetown University, estimates that the alcohol industry spent $2 billion on advertising in the media during 2005. Take into account other forms of promotion, such as product placement, Internet advertising, and sponsorships, and that figure jumps to approximately $6 billion during 2005. It should be noted that this figure was calculated based on an estimate from the Federal Trade Commission that states the alcohol industry spends approximately three times as much on total promotions as it does on media advertising.

The alcohol industry says that it does not broadcast ads for beer and wine during programs where more than half the viewers are under 21. Yet teens frequently watch programs broadcast after 9 P.M., which are supposedly aimed at adults.

Sporting events are also popular among teens. The group Common Sense Media analyzed 6,000 commercials that occurred during 60 National Football League games. Three hundred of those commercials were for alcohol. In fact, a 2008 report by the Marin Institute found that Anheuser-Bush has invested $250 million in ads during the Super Bowl over the past 20 years. Also, the Drug-Free Action

Alliance reported that in 2009, young people in Ohio found that beer commercials during the Super Bowl were among their favorite commercials.

At Georgetown University, the Center on Alcohol Marketing and Youth (CAMY) found that teens were increasingly exposed to alcohol advertising on television between 2001 and 2005. In a 2004 study, the organization also found that 66 percent of youth exposure to alcohol ads on the radio occurred during programming for young people between the ages of 12 and 18.

However, it is worth noting that exposure to alcohol commercials has dropped. According to the organization Campaign for a Commercial-Free Childhood, by 2007 only 6 percent of alcohol advertisements were on television shows where the youth audience was at least 30 percent.

The hidden message

Commercials for distilled spirits, such as whiskey, gin, and vodka, do not appear on American TV, yet commercials for beer and wine do. This creates a mistaken assumption that there is little risk involved in drinking beer or wine. In fact, all these products are alcoholic beverages, and they all have similar effects on the mind and body.

The various pre-mixed beverages that appear on the market every now and then may cause the most confusion. For example, in the 1980s, the alcohol industry began heavily marketing wine coolers via TV commercials.

Coolers are blends of wine and ingredients such as fruit juice that hide the taste of alcohol. They have a lower alcohol percentage than wine (6 percent compared with more than 13 percent for most wines). However, the average cooler bottle holds at least twice as much liquid as a wine glass, so the amount of alcohol in one serving is about the same. In other words, coolers are alcoholic beverages in every sense of the word, although many kids don't know that.

Wine coolers represent a far smaller portion of the alcohol market than beer. Beer commercials often use themes and images that kids find especially appealing. Some commercials show rugged-looking men and women scaling mountain cliffs or racing bikes over the roughest terrain. These ads may send a "hidden" message that drinking beer makes the viewer strong and tough.

Other commercials use sex appeal. Of course, most teenagers understand that drinking beer does not make boys suddenly attractive to beautiful women. Yet the question is: Do clever ads appeal to one's good sense—or to one's emotions?

The placement of alcohol commercials is an issue too. Kids tend to be fans of sports and music programs, many of which have alcohol sponsors. Advertisers build on kids' loyalty to their favorite stars, and transfer that appeal to the product they are advertising.

A 1994 study in the *American Journal of Public Health* reported an interesting connection between ads and what kids actually thought about drinking. The kids who were most aware of beer advertising were more likely to have favorable notions of drinking, and to express their intention to drink. The authors concluded that "alcohol advertising may pre-dispose young people to drinking."

In a 2006 study published in the *Archives of Pediatrics and Adolescent Medicine,* the authors found that exposure to alcohol advertising influenced the probability of drinking. According to the report, for each advertising dollar per capita spent, there was a 3 percent increase in youth drinking.

Not just TV

College campuses have one feature in common with popular TV shows—a mixed age group. While most freshmen, sophomores, and juniors are underage, the typical college also enrolls many graduate students, enough to make up a sizable market for advertisers. This provides an "in" for advertisers and promoters, who are legally entitled to advertise to the over-21 set. Brewers and beer distributors were spending $20 million a year on marketing to colleges in the 1990s, much of it on sponsorship of sporting events. However, by 2001, the majority of colleges told a National Collegiate Athletic Association survey that they no longer accepted alcohol ads at sporting events.

The growth of the Internet has provided another channel for alcohol marketing to reach kids. Brewers and distillers have put up some of the most exciting Web sites, with video, sound effects, interactive games, and product promotions.

WHAT SHOULD GOVERNMENT DO?

The government takes a much lower profile with alcohol advertising than it does with tobacco. One reason is that tobacco is harmful to all users, while alcohol may be used safely by some people.

Now and then, however, public-interest groups have called on the government to get involved. That happened in 1996, after the distilled spirits industry dropped its voluntary ban on TV and radio ads. The industry's Distilled Spirits Council (DISCUS) claimed that current practices discriminated against their companies in favor of beer brewers and wine manufacturers.

Their decision caused a public uproar. Hundreds of public-interest groups appealed to the Federal Communications Commission to intervene, and bills were proposed in Congress. In the end, most broadcasters refused the ads, and the voluntary ban remains in effect.

"COUNTERATTACK"

Given the apparent success of anti-smoking ads, some activists have begun calling for alcohol counteradvertising. They want to show ads that feature cool kids having fun *without* alcohol. According to a 2002 study by the National Institute on Alcohol Abuse and Alcoholism (NIAAA), "There is an increasing body of literature that suggests that alcohol counteradvertising is effective in reducing the alcohol consumption of teenagers and young adults."

THE ALCOHOL INDUSTRY'S VIEW

The alcohol industry consistently denies that it targets the under-21 age group, claiming that it does not want to waste money appealing to people who cannot legally buy their products. In March 2003, a spokesperson for DISCUS said, "Advertising, whether someone is of age or not, affects what they might choose to drink, not whether they drink."

Some independent observers agree. In 1997, an article appeared in *Priorities,* a reputable journal that sometimes takes controversial stands on public-health issues. The title of the article says it all: "Alcohol Advertising Does Not Promote Underage Drinking." The author claims that public fears that TV ads lead to teen alcohol abuse have not been backed up by research. He prefers to rely on the natural skepticism of young people as a defense against any hidden messages in the ads. He even speculates that advertising bans could backfire, since some kids seem to resent any attempt by grownups to "tell them what to do."

IT'S UP TO YOU

The controversy over alcohol advertising probably will be around for a long time to come, but the bottom line for teens is simple. Go ahead and laugh at the funny commercial—just don't forget all the facts you are learning about the very real risks of underage drinking. When the time comes for you to decide, remember that it is not cool to let anyone else make your decision for you, whether that is a real-life friend or an animated puppet on the TV screen.

See also: Drinking on College Campuses

■ ALCOHOL, HISTORY OF

Throughout recorded history, and probably long before, people have been making and drinking alcoholic beverages. Historians do not know where they were first discovered, but it is easy to guess how it might have happened.

Wild fruits, berries, and honey exposed to the air in warm weather naturally ferment—the sugar turns to alcohol and carbon dioxide. The yeast that helps the process along is floating in the air. For primitive people, food was always scarce. Sooner or later, some cave dwellers would have been willing to try a concoction they discovered in the woods that looked, smelled, and tasted spoiled. Almost every primitive people ever encountered has brewed beer or made wine. In the entire world, only the Polynesians and the Native Americans of the present-day United States and Canada did not discover and use alcohol on their own.

Once people invented writing and the arts, the record became clearer. Every ancient civilization left behind written evidence of alcoholic beverages.

The earliest civilizations in the ancient Near East, from Egypt to Mesopotamia, brewed beer from grains. Enterprising people sold the beverage in taverns, but rulers often distributed it free to citizens during religious festivals. Artists painted brewing scenes on walls and pottery. Archeologists have even found traces (tiny amounts) of beer still clinging to 5,000-year-old clay pitchers.

Ancient Hindu books from almost that far back tell about mead, a wine made from honey. Chinese people under the Shang dynasty more than 3,000 years ago drank beer, and may have drunk grape wine as well. In Mexico and Peru, long before the Spanish conquest, beer was made from corn. In Africa, grains, fruits, honey, and palm sap were used as raw materials for beer and wine.

Winemaking has been around for many thousands of years. But for most of history, beer was the most popular drink; in many countries, including the United States, it still is. The raw materials for beer—mainly grains, such as barley or corn—were much more common than grapes. Also, beer was quicker to make and easier to store.

Until the time of the Greeks, wine was considered an elite product, used in sacrifices to the gods or on ceremonial occasions by kings and their associates. By the time of the Romans, however, farmers were growing grapevines all across the Roman and Persian Empires. When the early Christian Church adopted wine for its central sacrament, wine had become perhaps the most popular alcoholic beverage. However, most people drank wine (naturally 8 to 12 percent alcohol) diluted by 50 percent with water.

Distilled spirits or liquors are a more recent invention. They do not occur naturally and did not become common until the late Middle Ages—after around A.D. 1200. These beverages, with their much higher alcohol content, caused many social problems and helped change the way many people viewed alcohol.

HISTORICAL USES

As far as historians can tell, people used—and abused—alcohol in the past in some of the same ways as they do today: for relaxation, to bring people together at social and religious events and celebrations, to give people "courage" to face unavoidable tasks, and to drown out sorrows and failures.

Alcohol was also used for medicinal purposes in ancient times, much more so than today. Doctors prescribed it to deaden pain when few other painkillers were known or available. Sumerian and Egyptian doctors wrote down recipes for beer-and-herb mixtures as treatments for various ailments.

Alcoholic beverages may have supplied much-needed nutrition as well. Early beer, less refined than today's, may have contained more starch and other nutrients; besides, beer can be stored easily and preserved for times of scarcity, as during the winter in northern regions. Today's alcoholic beverages, however, are a poor supply of nutrition.

Alcoholic beverages were also widely used as libations, poured offerings to the gods, often including special gods and goddesses of beer and wine. The Bible records that Moses provided for daily libations of wine in the Temple.

Large quantities of wine or beer were also handed out and consumed at religious or civic festivals, where drunkenness and wild dancing was sometimes considered holy. It was a way for people to achieve ecstasy and unite with the spirit world. The notorious bacchanalias, festivals to the wine god Bacchus, eventually became so destructive that the Roman Senate banned them from all of Italy.

Alcohol abuse as known today was also known to the ancient world. Literature from all over the world condemned drunkenness as a cause of immorality and violence; Bible stories about Noah and Lot are good examples. Stories and poetry sometimes depicted people who would today be called alcohol dependent or **alcoholics,** and ancient doctors knew about the health dangers of alcohol abuse.

Nevertheless, alcohol was rarely considered a major problem for society as a whole until the spread of cheap distilled spirits (mostly gin) in Europe in the 1600s and 1700s. Before then, drunkenness had usually been confined to special occasions, or kept hidden in people's homes. But in the growing cities of the early modern era, with their large, crowded populations, private behavior became everybody's business. Many people accustomed to beer, with its low alcohol content, could not handle the 45-percent alcohol content of gin and other distilled spirits.

As a result of the perceived harm to families and communities, a **temperance movement** began to emerge in England in the 18th century, centered on the independent churches. The movement advocated a "temperate" or moderate use of alcohol.

In England's American colonies, rum from the West Indies was popular, along with gin and whiskey. As in England, many American civic and church leaders began to preach against the abuse of alcohol—or even against its use in any amount. This was the start of what became the **prohibition** movement, an organized ban on the drinking of any alcohol.

LAWS CONTROLLING ALCOHOL USE AND PROHIBITION

Public laws and regulations to control the use and abuse of alcohol are almost as old as the beverages themselves. The famous Hammurabi Code, a series of laws issued by the Babylonian King Hammurabi around 1800 B.C., included measures such as fixing prices and controlling the sale of alcohol by taverns. In ancient Egypt, priests preached against overdrinking.

When the drinking of alcohol outside of religious occasions began to spread in ancient China, the government tried to impose prohibition, but it was never successfully enforced. Various rulers of ancient Persia, Greece, and Rome also tried to control or limit alcohol abuse.

Some of the major world religions have banned alcohol among their followers, though they have not always succeeded in enforcing the ban. For example, Buddhism has advised against alcohol since its start 2,500 years ago, yet alcohol is still widely used among the Buddhist peoples of south and east Asia. In India, the Hindu faith teaches that alcohol is impure. But despite the appeals for prohibition by Mahatma Gandhi and other leaders, only members of the elite Brahmin caste generally abstain from alcohol.

The Koran, the sacred text of the Muslim religion, strictly bans all alcohol. That ban has probably been the most successful prohibition effort in history. Alcohol is not easy to find in some Arab countries to this day. Even so, drinking is not unknown in most Muslim countries and is widespread in some.

In the modern world, nearly every country has laws to control the production, sale, and consumption of alcohol, to ensure a source of steady tax income for the government as well as to control and limit abuses. These practices began in England in the mid-1700s, when the government passed many laws to restrict the times and places that gin could be sold. The laws raised taxes on gin and tried to dilute its alcohol content. These measures were largely successful; England went back to its beer- and ale-drinking traditions, which it preserves to the present day.

The most famous attempt to limit drinking was the Eighteenth, or Prohibition, Amendment to the U.S. Constitution, passed in 1919. That "great experiment" is discussed in the entry on "Law and Drinking."

PRODUCTION OF ALCOHOL

Manufacturers all over the world offer a huge, confusing variety of alcoholic beverages for sale. Despite all those labels, all the products fall into only three basic categories: wine, beer, and liquor, or distilled spirits.

Wine

Wine (typically around 12 or 13 percent alcohol) is usually made from grapes, but other fruits can be used as well. (Apple cider is, strictly speaking, a kind of wine.) Winemakers use thousands of different grape varieties, which all derive from the same species of grape. Most of the grape's juice is naturally white: The color in red and rosé wines comes primarily from the skin.

DID YOU KNOW?

One Drink Equals . . .

12 ounces of beer (12-ounce bottle or can)
12 ounces of wine cooler (standard bottle)
5 ounces of wine (standard wine glass)
3 ounces of sherry or port (small wine glass)
1.5 ounces of brandy (standard shot glass)
1.5 ounces of 80-proof liquor (standard shot glass)
1 ounce of 120-proof liquor (two-thirds standard shot glass)
1.5–3 ounces of liqueur (check the label!)

Source: Indiana Prevention Resource Center, 2004.

Grapes are harvested, crushed, and poured into vats or barrels, where natural **fermentation,** a natural process in which sugar chemically turns into alcohol, takes place due to yeast in the grapes; extra sugar and yeast are sometimes added. During fermentation, much of the sugar turns to alcohol and carbon dioxide, which is usually allowed to evaporate.

Alcohol is toxic to yeast, so fermentation is a self-limiting process: It stops as soon as the alcohol reaches a concentration of 10 to 15 percent, which can happen over a few days or up to several weeks, depending on the type of wine. Sparkling wines, such as champagne, go through a second fermentation in the bottle, with sugar and yeast added to produce more carbon dioxide. Fortified wines, such as sherry and port, have brandy added to them to increase the percentage of alcohol, to as much as 23 percent. Liqueurs, or aperitifs, are sweet heavy wines to which herbs and other ingredients, such as quinine, are added for flavor. Wine coolers are carbonated blends of white wine and citrus juices.

Not long ago, France was the largest producer of wine in the world, followed by Italy, with French wines regarded as the best. But with the growth of globalization and the spread of technology, many other countries and regions have become major producers and exporters of wine, including California in the United States, several South American and eastern European countries, South Africa, and Australia.

Fact Or Fiction?

In France, where drinking wine with meals is an honored part of the culture, there is no alcoholism.

The Facts: Research proves this statement false. There are about two million alcoholics in France, according to recent research, roughly the same percentage of the population as in the United States. With so many people abusing alcohol, France suffers many of the alcohol-related problems Americans do: More than one third of all motor vehicle crash deaths, a quarter of suicides, and about one half of all homicides involve the beverage. It is interesting to note that French people have been drinking less wine in recent years, maybe because of campaigns aimed at kids with the message, "How do you look when you're drunk?"

Beer

Beer (ranging from 4 to more than 6 percent alcohol) can be made from any cereal grain, most often barley but also wheat, rice, or corn, or from starchy roots such as sweet potatoes. Unlike the sugar in grapes, the starch in grain does not ferment on its own. It needs to be turned into sugar by a process called **malting.**

For malting, the grain is first allowed to germinate in water (the seeds begin to grow into tiny plants). The germinated grain, or *malt,* is then cracked (separated from the husk), dried, and mashed into hot water, where it turns into sugar.

Brewers then add **hops,** an aromatic plant, for flavor, color, and aroma. Finally, they add yeast to promote fermentation of the sugar into alcohol. Fermentation can take up to several months.

Brewers produce various types of beer and ale (a type of beer) using different techniques. They can use different grains as raw material; add a variety of unmalted grains and vary the water temperature during the mashing step; use different types of yeast during fermentation to control carbonation; add various flavoring ingredients just before bottling; and allow the product to age more or less in the bottle before refrigeration or sale. Draft beer is beer that is not pasteurized (heated to kill germs); it must be kept refrigerated throughout the distribution path, unlike pasteurized beer, which can be stored safely at room temperature.

Q & A

Question: Is there any alcohol in "nonalcoholic" beer, and is there any risk involved in drinking this product?

Answer: Nonalcoholic beers are made from alcoholic beer. The alcohol is removed through evaporation, but a small amount does remain in the product—up to one-half of 1 percent. For people without a history of alcohol abuse, there should not be any problem drinking a cold, tasty "near beer." However, for alcoholics, the smell of nonalcoholic beer may trigger cravings for the real beverage. A study reported in the November 1999 issue of *Alcoholism: Clinical and Experimental Research* found that olfactory cues (smells) can easily trigger cravings for alcohol.

Liquor

Liquors, or distilled spirits (with widely ranging alcohol content of up to 90 percent), are all produced by the same two-step technique. The process was discovered more than 2,000 years ago but did not become widely adopted until around the year A.D. 1600.

The first step is fermentation, usually with grains as the initial raw material. The second step is distillation, a process during which the distiller boils the fermented mash. The boiling yields a steam of alcohol and flavorings; the steam rises into another, cooler container, where it condenses back into liquor. Since much of the nonalcoholic liquid stays behind, the liquor has a much higher alcohol content.

Whiskeys are various grain liquors traditionally aged for a period of years in oak barrels. Slight differences in processing, and different alcohol percentages, account for the different tastes and textures. Bourbon is made largely from corn and aged in barrels that have been charred. Scotch is usually exposed to peat smoke. Rye is produced largely from rye grain, and corn liquor is produced mostly from corn.

Vodka, made from potatoes or grain, generally has the same alcohol content as whiskey (roughly 40–50 percent), but it is filtered through charcoal to remove color and taste. Gin is flavored with juniper berries. Brandy and cognac are distilled from grape wine. Rum is made from sugarcane or molasses, and tequila from the agave plant.

Every country and people in the world has its own variations of liquors, with different additives, mixers, and raw materials. The alcohol concentration can vary greatly, but is always much greater than that in beer or wine. In the United States, alcohol is labeled with its **proof,** which is twice its alcohol percentage by volume. In other words, liquor labeled as 80-proof is 40 percent alcohol by volume. Remember, that is more than *three times* as potent as most wines and *seven times* as potent as beer.

See also: Effects on the Body; Ethnicity and Alcohol; Law and Drinking, The

FURTHER READING
Gately, Iain. *Drink: A Cultural History of Alcohol.* New York: Gotham, 2009.
Holt, Mack. *Alcohol: A Social and Cultural History.* Gordonsville, Va.: Berg Publishers, 2006.
Lembeck, Harriet. *Grossman's Cyclopedia: The Concise Guide to Wines, Beers, and Spirits.* Philadelphia: Running Press, 2002.
Phillips, Roderick. *A Short History of Wine.* New York: Ecco, 2000.
Smith, Gregg. *Beer: A History of Suds and Civilization from Mesopotamia to Microbreweries.* New York: Avon, 1995.

■ ALCOHOL ABUSE, THE RISKS OF

Alcohol abuse refers to the potential "down side" or consequences of a drinking pattern that leads to **intoxication** or **addiction** causing one or more behavior problems. You have probably heard the expression "calculated risk." Most of the choices people make in life involve a price they have to pay if things go wrong. As teenagers leave childhood behind and begin to think and act like adults, they may find it useful to calculate, or think through, the benefits and risks of possible behaviors. Alcohol abuse is one of those behaviors.

The problem behaviors that can result from alcohol abuse can include failure to live up to your responsibilities; drinking under dangerous conditions; getting in frequent trouble with the law; and having alcohol-related problems with a spouse or friend.

Of course, people do not stop a hundred times a day to do the calculations. At any point in their lives, most people do what is routine. For example, adults who have mastered the art of drinking in moderation do not need to stop and think each time they have a glass of wine with dinner. Other adults, who have decided to abstain from any alcohol, do not bother to rethink the issue every time someone offers them a drink. And, unfortunately, **alcoholics** may feel powerless to change their unhealthy behavior patterns. Young people, however, who have not yet settled into regular behavior patterns, can learn about the risks and do their own calculations. They should be aware that the decisions they make can eventually become habits.

THE RISK OF INJURY

According to the Centers for Disease Control and Prevention (CDC), more than 150,000 Americans die every year from trauma to the body—in other words, injury. Trauma is the leading cause of death for people aged one to 44. Millions more suffer nonfatal injuries—one out of three individuals, according to the CDC. Sometimes it seems as if the world is one big booby trap, ready to go off without warning.

In almost every case, physicians or emergency staff can find an immediate cause for these deaths: for example, a vehicle crash, fire, poisoning, or deliberate act of violence. However, too often, the real underlying cause is alcohol use or alcohol abuse, meaning a pattern of drinking that results in at least one of these behaviors: failure to fulfill major responsibilities; drinking in dangerous situations, for example, when driving; having alcohol-related legal problems; having alcohol-related relationship problems.

According to the CDC, excessive alcohol use is the third leading life-style-related cause of death in the United States. A 2008 fact sheet produced by the CDC indicates that 33.3 percent of people who committed suicide tested positive for alcohol. The state of Virginia reports that between 2003 and 2006, 39 percent of homicide victims had alcohol in their system. Twenty-two percent of homicide victims had a blood alcohol content of .08 or greater at the time of death. The National Institute of Justice estimates that 14 percent of homicide, or attempted homicide, victims had alcohol in their system at the time of the crime.

The problem is a long-standing one. According to a 1989 "Alcohol Alert" from the National Institute of Alcohol Abuse and Alcoholism, surveys also showed a high percentage of injuries involving people with high BALs. Intoxicated individuals caused some 40–50 percent of motor vehicle fatalities (deaths), 25–35 percent of nonfatal motor vehicle injuries, 64 percent of fires and burns, 48 percent of frostbite and hypothermia (very low body temperature, generally resulting from passing out or sleeping outdoors in cold weather), and 20 percent of suicides.

Furthermore, most studies show that the alcohol-related injuries tend to be the more serious ones. The reasons are clear. Alcohol, even at moderate levels, can weaken people's judgment, slow down their reaction times, and make them clumsy and uncoordinated. That is why no supervisor with any sense allows a worker to operate dangerous machinery while under the influence of alcohol.

Q & A

Question: We know that people who operate machinery in the workplace should not drink. What about operating machinery for recreation? For example, what about boating?

Answer: More than half of all recreational boating deaths involve alcohol. According to the U.S. Coast Guard, "a boat operator with a blood alcohol concentration above .10 is 10 times more likely to be killed in a boating accident than a boater with a zero blood alcohol concentration." A little bit of alcohol may actually be more dangerous for boaters than for automobile drivers. Sun, wind, noise, vibration, and boat motion can enhance the effects of alcohol. You should be alert when operating *any* vehicle.

RISKS IN THE EMERGENCY ROOM

Being sober is no guarantee that you will always avoid injury. Also, people who have been drinking might become trauma victims through events beyond their control. But even if alcohol did not cause an injury, drinking entails an additional risk for those who are injured: It can get in the way of a doctor making a quick, accurate diagnosis.

When a trauma victim turns up at a hospital emergency room (ER) with a bruise on the forehead, slurred speech, and an unsteady gait, the medical staff would normally suspect a serious head injury. But when they get a strong whiff of alcohol as they approach the victim, they suddenly see a different picture. They should still check for serious injury, but in the real, high-pressure world of an ER, some staff might be tempted to lead the victim to a bed to "sleep it off" while they deal with other emergencies.

If a patient who has been drinking does *not* show signs of intoxication in the ER, that can be dangerous too. Alcohol does not mix well with many standard medications, including antibiotics and painkillers. If the patient is unconscious, confused, or fails to tell staff that he or she has been drinking, the wrong drug may be administered, with dangerous results.

THE RISK OF UNINTENDED DEATH

Some unlucky people are deathly allergic to even one peanut. Everyone else, fortunately, can eat as many as they could possibly want and still suffer no more than a bellyache. The reverse is true of alcohol. Almost no one is truly allergic to the substance, but *anyone* can get seriously ill or even die if he or she drinks too fast, too much, or in combination with certain other substances.

Binge drinking

Regular heavy drinking can be dangerous to your health. Binge drinking, when someone has five or more drinks on one occasion, is an injury waiting to happen. But **chugging,** drinking a large quantity in a short period of time, can kill.

As a general rule, the liver of an average person can metabolize, or break down, the alcohol in one drink in about an hour. People who drink more than one drink an hour, whether shots of whiskey or bottles of beer, are overloading their bloodstreams with alcohol. The more they put into their systems, the higher their blood alcohol level.

When your BAL goes above .08 (which may happen after just a few standard-sized drinks), you are considered unfit to drive in most states (although some people may be unfit to drive at lower levels too). As the level rises (and it surely does if you drink too fast), the toxic (poisonous) effects of alcohol on the brain and nervous system start to kick in. When your BAL hits .25, you lose your coordination, and you can easily choke on your own vomit if you are alone or if your drinking companions are also intoxicated and unable to help.

When you continue chugging, your BAL can rise above .30, when you could pass out. At .35, your breathing may stop; without immediate medical care to restore your breathing, you may die. At .40, even if your breathing can be restored, you may suffer permanent brain damage and slip into a coma.

You might think that once you pass out and can no longer continue drinking, you can never reach the deadly levels. Unfortunately, the BAL can keep rising even *after* you stop drinking, as the alcohol in your stomach continues to be absorbed into the bloodstream faster than your body can break it down. If your friends pour coffee into you, push you into a cold shower, or walk you around the room, you might feel a bit more alert, but none of those measures reduces the BAL and the damage it can cause. If someone you know passes out after chugging, you should seek immediate medical attention.

Fact Or Fiction?

"If my friend has had so much to drink he's passed out, he can be revived if I make him drink lots of coffee."

The Facts: Wrong. Coffee may help keep your friend awake, but it will have no impact on his blood alcohol level. If he has had so much alcohol to drink that he passes out, he may be in danger. If you are reasonably sober, keep a very close watch to make sure he continues to breathe normally, and make sure he's lying on his side or upright to keep him from choking on his own vomit. If you are not in a condition to monitor your friend, you should get help from someone who can.

Chugging

Chugging is drinking a large amount of alcohol in as short a time as possible. It is relatively rare among adults, but all too common among the underage. Underage drinkers are more likely to engage in the activity for several reasons, apart from lack of experience and lack of knowledge. Teenagers know they are not allowed to buy alcohol when attending a party, concert, or sporting event. To compensate, some kids chug down several drinks before they arrive at their destination, as if their stomachs were fuel tanks that they can tap as needed in the course of an evening.

But it doesn't work that way at all. Instead, *all* the alcohol is absorbed into the blood in a matter of an hour or so. Instead of a steady high, these young drinkers can expect a brief roller-coaster ride, with extreme intoxication followed by physical or mental collapse.

Kids who feel insecure may try to impress friends with their ability to hold their liquor. And kids who want to be accepted by a club or fraternity—or by any crowd of other kids—may calculate that the goal is worth accepting the challenge to chug. If they understood that the risk is brain damage or death, would the calculation come out the same?

Even modest amounts of alcohol can kill when combined with certain prescription or over-the-counter medications or with illicit drugs. At the very least, if you are fighting a bacterial infection, alcohol can make antibiotics lose their effect in your system, leading to a surge in the bacteria you are trying to fight. At the worst, alcohol can intensify the effects of certain other drugs, causing unpredictable damage to vital body systems.

When mixing drugs and alcohol, a little bit of knowledge can be a dangerous thing. A friend may tell you that mixing alcohol with a particular drug gives you a stronger high and can't harm you. Perhaps your friend has done it once or twice and lived to tell the tale. But remember, before any drug can be legally sold, it is tested on thousands of people for a period of several years, and every bad reaction is carefully recorded. Unless your friend's concoction has undergone such scrutiny, it cannot be trusted. Play it safe and avoid taking unnecessary risks.

DOMESTIC ABUSE

Domestic abuse, the regular mistreatment of one family member or romantic partner by another, is one of the more heartbreaking phenomena often associated with problem drinking. A study in the December 1999 *New England Journal of Medicine* reported that alcohol abuse was the greatest single risk factor causing injuries to female victims of domestic violence. But the problem goes well beyond the headline-grabbing crimes of violence. Abuse can include frightening verbal assaults, insults and unfair criticism, denial of affection, broken promises, poor supervision, lack of support, or neglect.

This is still the case. In a 2006 study published in *Alcoholism: Clinical and Experimental Research,* the authors found that weekly heavy drinking was significantly related to domestic violence among white and Hispanic soldiers in the army. In a 2008 study in *Addictive Behaviors,* researchers found that the frequency of alcohol use was related to men engaging in domestic violence. Women who drank more were also more likely to experience domestic violence from their partners.

Child abuse is a growing problem. According to the Administration for Children and Families, in 2006 an estimated 905,000 children were found to be victims of neglect or abuse. Children from birth to one year of age had the highest rate of victimization, at 24.4 percent of children abused per 100,000 children studied of the same age group.

Among all age groups, 64.1 percent suffered from neglect, 16 percent suffered physical abuse, and 8.8 percent suffered sexual abuse.

In 1999, the National Center on Addiction and Substance Abuse (CASA) at Columbia University stated that alcohol and drug abuse among parents are the most important causes of the rise in child abuse and neglect in recent years. The center found that parents who abuse drugs or alcohol are 2.7 times more likely to abuse their kids, and more than 4 times more likely to neglect them. The NCCANI reported in 2003 that an earlier (1989) study found that alcohol and drug abuse by parents were involved in some 70 percent of child neglect cases in many urban areas.

Substance abuse is not generally the *only* cause of these problems. Other personal or social factors are often involved too, but alcohol makes the problems worse and harder to resolve. A parent whose time and money are devoted to heavy drinking is less likely to carry out his or her responsibilities to spouse and children.

Parental neglect and alcohol abuse are related in another way. Even the best of parents may not be able to protect their children in every situation. However, parents who abuse alcohol are less able to provide their teenage kids with supervision or attention, and poor parental supervision is an important cause of teenage alcohol abuse.

NOT AN EQUAL-OPPORTUNITY DRUG: WOMEN AND ALCOHOL ABUSE

In the past, researchers found that, for Americans as a whole, men are twice as likely as women to suffer from alcohol abuse or alcohol dependency. This gap may be disappearing, if behavior among teenagers is any guide. A 2007 study found that male and female 12th graders are just as likely to drink (47.1 percent v. 41.4 percent) and have been drunk (31.7 percent v. 25.7 percent).

Some researchers say that gender equality is in part responsible for this change. Many girls now believe that they do not have to follow old-fashioned ideas about "feminine" behavior. Some may think, "If boys can do it, even though it's illegal and risky, why can't we girls?" Unfortunately, nature is not always fair. Behaviors that are harmful for one gender may be even more harmful for the other. Alcohol abuse is one of those, and the female gender suffers the most.

If a boy and a girl drink the same quantity of alcohol, the girl's BAL is higher, for at least three reasons. To begin with, girls tend to be smaller than boys, at any age group, and body size influences how much alcohol can be safely imbibed. Secondly, boys have more active stomach enzymes, protein chemicals in the stomach that speed up chemical reactions, such as breaking down alcohol before it can be absorbed into the bloodstream. Finally, according to the National Institute on Alcohol Abuse and Alcoholism, even when a man and a woman have the same body size, the man has higher body water content, which dilutes the alcohol to some degree.

The higher BAL has two dangerous consequences: the girl becomes intoxicated sooner than the boy, and her health is more likely to suffer. On the average, American women live several years longer than men. But women alcohol abusers do not benefit from the same advantage—they have higher death rates than male alcohol abusers for several different alcohol-related problems, including liver disease, unintentional injuries, and suicide.

In addition, too much alcohol can upset the delicate balance of hormones that control a woman's reproductive system. This can cause menstrual periods to be irregular or painful, or even to stop altogether. Among pregnant women, it can cause miscarriage. Among older women, it can cause premature menopause.

Heavy drinkers, or people who have five or more drinks per occasion at least five different times a month, often lose calcium, a vital nutrient for bones and all body cells. Alcohol seems to upset the chemical systems that distribute the mineral through the body. Calcium actually drains away from bone tissue and is expelled in urine. This happens with men as well as women, but the consequences seem to be worse for females. Because women have a greater natural risk of osteoporosis, a disease of the bones that can lead to weakness and fractures, the additional damage caused by alcohol can make the difference between a manageable condition and crippling pain.

Some of the social consequences of alcohol abuse—whether by men *or* by women—fall more heavily on women too. Such consequences may include spousal abuse, rape, and unplanned or unprotected sex, which in turn can cause unwanted pregnancy and sexually transmitted diseases.

Alcohol in large, persistent quantities can be devastating to women. On the other hand, *small* amounts of alcohol (one or two drinks a day) may help older women produce estrogen, the basic female hormone, according to a study reported by the National Institute on Alcohol Abuse and Alcoholism in 2001. As a result, moderate women drinkers have a *lower* risk than nondrinkers for osteoporosis and heart disease.

TEENS SPEAK

Girls Are Different, Sometimes

"The worst part is, I finally find a boy I really like, and then we have to break up," Carolynn says. "My parents never tell me what to do, but this time they got scared. And the truth is, I had to agree they're right."

Carolynn had just started her junior year. She was feeling very mature and self-confident after volunteering at a camp for disabled kids, and she was starting to hang out with a nice ("really cute") guy.

The only problem was that Matthew and his friends like to drink. "Every Friday night they get together at Matthew's brother's apartment and work their way through all these six-packs. I told him, 'Sure I drink beer.' But all I ever have is one glass, at my father's barbecues."

That Friday night Carolynn and another girl started in with the guys. "After the second beer I was really buzzed," she remembers. "I was the only one; everyone thought it was funny." She thinks the other girl stopped after two, but Carolynn wanted to keep up with Matthew—"I can do anything a boy can," she remembers thinking.

What she didn't know is that alcohol works faster on women, and it works faster on smaller people. Carolynn is five foot four and weighs 115 pounds; Matthew is a hefty five ten and a half. When you take weight and sex into account, she really had two drinks for every one of his.

"I wound up vomiting in Matthew's lap just before I conked out," she says. She was incoherent when Matthew handed her over to her parents; her mother insisted on taking a picture so she could see herself the next morning. "It's a picture I'll never forget," she promises.

THE SOCIAL COSTS

Economists have tried to calculate the economic cost to society of alcohol abuse. Unfortunately, hospitals and insurance companies do not always keep separate tabulations of illnesses and injuries that are caused, or partly caused, by alcohol abuse; thus, the calculations are really estimates, or educated guesses.

Also, it is impossible to measure how much more productive alcohol abusers could be if they overcame their drinking problems. Nevertheless, in 2000, the U.S. Department of Health and Human Services felt sure enough about the facts to estimate that the cost of alcohol abuse to the U.S. economy in 1998 was $185 billion. The largest component was lost earnings and production in the workplace, figured at $134 billion. Medical costs came to nearly $19 billion, not including $7.5 billion for treatment programs. Alcohol-related crime cost $6.3 billion, while alcohol-related motor vehicle crashes cost $5.7 billion.

How do these costs add up? For starters, alcohol abusers cost employers four times the average amount in sickness and injury benefits. They also have double the normal rate of absence from work—9 percent of heavy drinkers miss work due to hangovers, according to the National Council on Alcohol and Drug Dependency, while 6 percent actually go to work drunk. There is no way to calculate the effects of intoxicated employees on coworker morale and client relations.

If these figures are correct, the annual cost to society is approximately $14,000 for each problem drinker (based on a total of 13 million, according to the 2001 National Household Survey on Drug Abuse). That's an expensive habit.

THE HEALTH COSTS

A 2004 report by the CDC estimated how many deaths could be attributed to the use or abuse of alcohol and the costs associated with those deaths. According to the report, in 2001 an estimated 75,766 alcohol-related deaths occurred. Forty-six percent of these were from chronic, or long-term, conditions, while 54 percent were from acute causes (for example, alcohol poisoning, suicide, homicide, accidents).

WEIGH YOUR RISKS

The short-term benefits of alcohol may be obvious to teenagers experimenting with alcoholic beverages. Alcohol can help people relax and have a good time, and may make kids feel accepted and part of the group. The risks, however, are often not immediately apparent. Smart, mature teenagers will try to weigh the present and future factors together when making their decisions about this important part of life.

See also: Alcohol and Disease; Alcohol and Violence; Children of Alcoholics; Drinking and Drugs; Effects on the Body; Sexual Behavior and Alcohol, Withdrawal

FURTHER READING

Kuhn, Cynthia, Scott Swartzwelder, and Wilkie Wilson. *Just Say Know: Talking with Kids about Drugs and Alcohol.* New York: Norton, 2002.

——. *Buzzed.* New York: W.W. Norton, 2008.

Sweeney, Donal F. *The Alcohol Blackout: Walking, Talking, Unconscious & Lethal.* Surrey, U.K.: Mnemosyne Press, 2004.

Volkmann, Chris, and Toren Volkmann. *From Binge to Blackout: A Mother and Son Struggle with Teen Drinking.* New York: New American Library, 2006.

Windle, Michael T. *Alcohol Use among Adolescents.* Thousand Oaks, Calif.: Sage Publications, 1999.

■ ALCOHOL AND DEPRESSION

Relationship between the use of alcohol and depression. This established relationship between alcohol and depression is a complex one. Alcohol use influences depression, and depression influences alcohol use. The relationship is cyclical, each element influencing the other. Research shows that this vicious cycle between alcohol and depression is stronger for women than for men.

MENTAL HEALTH AND ALCOHOL

Researchers from the National Alliance on Mental Illness (NAMI) estimate that 15 million adults suffer from major depressive disorder. Further, the Alliance estimates that 5.2 million adults have both a mental health and a **substance abuse** disorder such as those associated with drugs or alcohol.

The CDC estimate that 47.9 percent of all people age 18 and older are current regular drinkers. This translates into more than 102 million adults. Also, more men than women drink—57.4 versus 39.2 percent, respectively.

The authors of a 2009 report in *Preventing Chronic Disease,* published by the CDC, estimate that adults who had at least one major depressive episode (MDE) in the past year were more likely to drink heavily than those without an MDE.

Q & A

Question: Can drinking alcohol in moderate amounts help reduce the likelihood of becoming depressed?

Answer: There is conflicting evidence about this question. A 2005 study in the *American Journal of Public Health* found no difference in depression between those who did not drink alcohol and those who engaged in moderate levels of drinking. However, another study in a 2005 issue of the *American Journal of Public Health* found that moderate drinkers (having one to two drinks a day) had lower levels of depression when compared to nondrinkers and heavy drinkers. The thinking is that drinking some alcohol reduces stress and corresponding depression. Those who do not drink at all are said to be more stressed and therefore more depressed. Those who drink too much are said to have other very significant problems, with alcohol contributing to those problems.

A COMPLICATED RELATIONSHIP

The relationship between alcohol and depression is complicated. Alcohol use and abuse is a way to temporarily escape from one's problems in an attempt to feel better. However, excessive alcohol use can create problems, which then can lead to depression.

Research shows that depression influences alcohol consumption. In a 2005 study published in the *Journal of Studies on Alcohol,* researchers examined patients who entered an alcohol-treatment program. They found that patients drink more frequently and more heavily at the beginning of treatment if they have high levels of depression. This is important to consider when treating alcoholism because patients are more likely to drop out of programs at the beginning. By assessing and treating depression at the start of an alcohol-treatment program, there is a better chance fewer clients will drop out. Additionally, given the established relationship between alcohol and depression, medical staff can better determine who may be more likely to drink heavily at the outset. The authors further found that alcohol use also influences later depression.

In a 2008 study in the *Journal of Clinical Psychiatry,* researchers examined the differences between depressed patients with and without

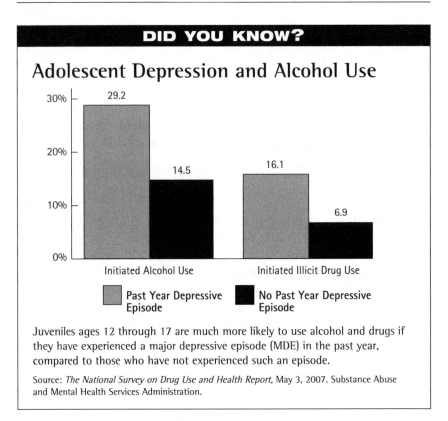

DID YOU KNOW?

Adolescent Depression and Alcohol Use

Juveniles ages 12 through 17 are much more likely to use alcohol and drugs if they have experienced a major depressive episode (MDE) in the past year, compared to those who have not experienced such an episode.

Source: *The National Survey on Drug Use and Health Report,* May 3, 2007. Substance Abuse and Mental Health Services Administration.

an alcohol disorder. The authors found that depressed patients with an alcohol disorder, compared to those without a disorder, were younger when they had their first episode of depression. These patients also had more depressive episodes and were younger when they had their first psychiatric hospitalization. Lastly, depressed patients with an alcohol disorder were younger when they first attempted suicide and had more suicide attempts.

Authors of another study in a 2006 issue of the *Canadian Journal of Psychiatry* provide similar findings. They state that people with depression are more than twice as likely to develop an alcohol disorder, compared to those who do not suffer with depression.

In a 2008 study in the *American Journal of Emergency Medicine,* the authors examined the relationship between alcohol and depression among patients in an emergency department in Los Angeles. The results show that patients with symptoms of depression are more likely to be at-risk, problem, or binge drinkers. Patients who were considered at-risk drinkers were 2.49 times more likely to report symptoms of depression. Problem and binge drinkers were approximately twice as likely to report symptoms of depression, compared to those who did not have problems with alcohol.

In a study in Finland, researchers followed children from 1989 to 1996, and, for parts of the study, they asked about alcohol use and depression. Researchers collected information in 1989, 1993, and 1996. The authors of a 2002 paper in *Addictive Behaviors* used the data from the study in Finland to examine how depression and alcohol use influenced each other over time. The authors found that children who were clinically depressed in 1993 *and* 1996 were almost four times more likely to be heavy alcohol users in 1996, compared to other children. Children were only twice as likely to be heavy alcohol users in 1996 if they were found to be clinically depressed in either 1993 *or* 1996. The authors reported that, in girls, thoughts of committing suicide preceded heavy alcohol use. This relationship between thoughts of suicide and drinking was not present for boys. Similarly, low self-esteem was a predictor of alcohol use for girls. People with low self-esteem are more likely to be depressed than those with high self-esteem.

A 2008 study in the *Journal of Studies on Alcohol and Drugs* also followed adolescents over time to examine the relationship between alcohol and depression. Researchers collected information about alcohol use at ages 16 and 18. Data about depression was collected at age 22. The authors found that problems stemming from alcohol use predicted depression at age 22. Alcohol consumption, on the other hand, was not related to future depression. The authors suggest that it is the problems that result from alcohol use, as opposed to the amount of alcohol one drinks, that lead to depression.

ALCOHOL USE, DEPRESSION, AND PARENTING STYLE

A 2007 study in the journal *Psychology of Addictive Behaviors* helps further illustrate the complex relationship between alcohol use and depression. The authors of this study examined how parenting styles and attachment to parents influenced both alcohol use and depression. The authors state that the type of relationship someone has with a parent is linked to both depression and drinking behavior. In this study, the authors examined how parenting style influenced the parent/child relationship. They then examined how the parent/child relationship influenced depression, which then influenced problematic drinking. Children who had fathers with an authoritative parenting style were less depressed than those whose fathers were permissive. Children with lower levels of depression were then less likely to engage in problematic drinking. Although the father's parenting style had an effect on depression and on subsequent alcohol abuse, the child/mother relationship did not have an effect.

ALCOHOL USE, DEPRESSION, AND DIFFERENT GROUPS

A 2009 study in *Addictive Behaviors* focused on the relationship between negative emotions and alcohol dependence among British Indian and white college students. The researchers wanted to see if the relationship between alcohol and depression differed between the groups. Although there was a relationship between alcohol and depression for white students, there was not one for the British Indian students. However, the study was designed in a way that measured both anxiety and depression as negative emotions. Therefore, in this case, the authors did not conclusively demonstrate an alcohol use-depression relationship.

GENDER, ALCOHOL, AND DEPRESSION

Men and women differ in their patterns of alcohol use and experiences with depression. According to a 2008 report by the CDC, women are significantly more likely to experience depression than men. Approximately 6.7 percent of women over the age of 12 were depressed in 2005 and 2006. Only 4 percent of men were depressed in the same time period. A 2006 report by the CDC showed that for every 100,000 women, 27.8 were hospitalized for depression between 2002 and 2004. However, only 14.5 per 100,000 men were hospitalized. Other data reveal the same findings, that significantly more women than men experience depression.

A 2002 study in the *Canadian Journal of Psychiatry* examined the role of depression on alcohol use for both men and women. The data came from a Canadian survey where respondents are interviewed over a period of several years. The authors found that depression played no role in subsequent alcohol use for men and women who do not drink. In other words, people with depression were no more likely to start drinking than those without depression. However, the results were different when looking at men and women who do use alcohol. Researchers discovered that women with depression were more likely to become frequent heavy drinkers than those who were not depressed. This was not the case for men.

When measuring depression, researchers in a 2009 study found that women who are dependent on alcohol score significantly higher than men, as reported in the journal *Addictive Behaviors*. The authors believe this is an indication that women tend to experience more depressive symptoms than men. The findings indicate that there is a stronger relationship between depression and alcohol use for women than for men.

The authors of a 2009 study in the *Journal of Substance Abuse Treatment* also found that women with an alcohol problem demonstrate more depressive symptoms than men. They also discovered that alcohol-related impairment has a stronger relationship to depression than how often and how much someone drinks.

In yet another study, in Sweden, researchers collected data on depression over a 50-year period, between 1947 and 1997. These results, too, indicate that alcohol disorders create a risk for depression. In this last case, the relationship was present for men but not for women.

See also: Recovery and Treatment

FURTHER READING
Sher, Leo. *Comorbidity of Depression and Alcohol Use Disorders.* Hauppauge, N.Y.: Nova Science Publishers, 2009.
Tatarsky, Andrew. *Harm Reduction Psychotherapy: A New Treatment for Drug and Alcohol Problems.* New York: Jason Aronson Publishers, 2007.

■ ALCOHOL AND DISEASE

A disease is any impairment or injury to the normal function of an organism. Alcohol is such a potent substance that few organ or body systems are immune from its effects. Some of the effects described above are healthy, but most are not, especially those caused by heavy or abusive drinking. No doubt you have discovered in school, at home, and among your friends that when it comes to making decisions, facing challenges, and learning about new things, no situation, problem, or issue is ever all black or all white, all bad or all good. The same holds true for alcohol and your health.

There is good news and bad news about alcohol's effects on the body—especially on the heart, circulatory system (blood), and brain. First, the good news.

RECENT RESEARCH ON ALCOHOL AND ADULTS

In recent years, some scientists who study alcohol's effects on people's health have gathered evidence that suggests that moderate drinking for adults—about two to three drinks a day for men, one to two drinks for women—appears to reduce the risk of heart attacks and strokes. Moderate drinking appears to raise "good" cholesterol levels, inhibit blood clotting, increase blood flow, and reduce blood pressure—all factors that contribute to healthy hearts and brains. It may also decrease a person's chances of developing brain-related diseases such as Alzheimer's and Parkinson's.

It's not what's drunk, but when and how

Scientists first believed that drinking red wine in moderation, just a few times a week, was the most likely way to reap beneficial health effects. They based their theory, in part, on the fact that people in heavy wine-consuming countries, such as France, appeared to have fewer heart-related health problems than other populations, despite a diet high in animal fat.

In September 2003 a group of scientists reported in the journal *Nature* that red wine may have some particularly beneficial effects after all. They reported that **resveratrol,** a chemical found abundantly in red wine, had the effect of stimulating long life in yeast plants and might possibly be involved in preventing diseases of aging in humans as well.

In January 2003, the "drinking-in-moderation" theory was expanded dramatically when the results of Harvard's 12-year Health Professional's Follow-Up Study were published. Scientists analyzed the drinking habits and health histories of more than 37,000 male health professionals (doctors, dentists, optometrists, osteopaths, and veterinarians) for more than a decade.

They concluded that individuals who had one to two drinks at least three days a week lowered their risk of heart attack by 32 to 37 percent. Those who drank at that level on at least five days a week had the lowest risk. In contrast, those who drank once or twice a week lowered their risk of heart attack by only 16 percent, and people who didn't drink at all had an *increased* risk of heart attack.

In other words, these experts reported that drinking frequently, but in moderation, may be part of a healthy lifestyle. Does this mean everyone should start consuming up to 14 drinks a week? Not at all. These experts caution that people who do not now drink should not necessarily begin, given all the potential negative effects of drinking, in particular the risks for people who have never drunk or have stopped drinking in the past.

Studies about alcohol benefits may be biased

Researchers who study the benefits of alcohol focus almost exclusively on older, educated, professional white males who may naturally be inclined to take good care of themselves and who have better access to health education and preventive health care. In research terms, this is called a *built-in bias*. These characteristics make these people a select population group that cannot be fairly compared to other groups, especially young people, women, and those from a lower socioeconomic background.

When it comes to teenagers, for example, the brain—particularly the portions of the brain responsible for learning, memory, and decision making—continues to develop through young adulthood. And this younger "learning" brain is very sensitive to the damaging effects of alcohol.

Scientists have demonstrated in problem-solving situations that consuming the equivalent of just one drink can impair learning ability in young drinkers up to the age of 25. The same amount of alcohol may show no effect on older people's brains in similar situations. In other words, you and your brain (and for that matter, the rest of your body) may have a lot of growing to do before you can think about making "healthy drinking" a part of your life!

Moderate drinking is a relative term

Despite the evidence that moderate daily drinking may be good for one's health, this theory does not hold up for developing adolescents, teens, and young adults, whose brains and other organs are especially vulnerable to the effects of alcohol.

The phrase *moderate drinking* is a very relative term: That is to say, every individual reacts to alcohol uniquely. What's "moderate" for your parents or a friend may be excessive and damaging for you. In fact, many people who develop serious liver damage from drinking too much tell their doctors that they are only moderate drinkers and deny ever having been drunk.

Fact Or Fiction?

Men and women are not equal when it comes to drinking.

The Facts: This is true. Men who consume two to three drinks a day may reduce their risk for heart attack and stroke by as much as 37 percent. Yet women who consume two or more drinks a day may increase their risk of breast cancer by as much as 41 percent. Women drinkers also develop alcohol-related brain, heart, and liver damage much faster than comparable male drinkers, even when drinking less alcohol than men.

People who say alcohol "goes right to your head" (meaning, your brain) are right. At least, that's where you first feel the effects of alcohol. But alcohol also goes to every other organ and cell in your body. It uses your bloodstream to make the trip.

THE BLOODSTREAM: ALCOHOL'S SUPERHIGHWAY

Your body digests, or slowly breaks down, most of the food you eat into nutrients, which are absorbed by the body, and waste materials, which are eliminated.

Unlike food, alcohol is *not* digested. When you drink, alcohol passes directly into your bloodstream through the cells of your digestive tract. It begins its journey in your mouth and throat (where 5 percent of the alcohol in a drink enters the bloodstream within seconds), travels on to your stomach (where 25 percent is absorbed within minutes), and ends in your small intestine (where 70 percent is absorbed within an hour).

It takes from 30 minutes (on an empty stomach) to 60 minutes (on a full stomach) for all the alcohol in one drink to enter your bloodstream. Once alcohol is there, the heart circulates it, via your blood, to all parts of your body. The greatest amounts of alcohol go to those organs that receive the biggest supplies of blood—your brain, liver, and kidneys.

The largest of these organs, the liver, has the vital task of metabolizing, or breaking down, alcohol and removing it from your bloodstream quickly and efficiently. The liver can do this at the rate of about one drink an hour. If you consume more than one drink in an hour, the liver becomes overworked and cannot metabolize all the alcohol in your body.

The more you drink, and the more quickly you drink, the less efficiently your liver works. The result is that larger quantities of alcohol remain in your bloodstream for a longer time. Because alcohol travels to and affects all parts of your body, this type of drinking—too much, too quickly—can cause severe health problems for your body.

Occasional episodes of this type of drinking can cause minor, short-term health problems; but even one episode of chugging, or drinking one drink after another, can put you in the hospital. A regular pattern of overdrinking can have serious, long-term health consequences. Take a brief look at some of these potential short- and long-term health problems, starting with the gastrointestinal (GI) tract.

ALCOHOL AND YOUR GI TRACT

Alcohol irritates the lining of your mouth, throat, esophagus (the "tube" in which food travels), stomach, and intestines. Possible short-term or minor health problems include nausea, vomiting, diarrhea, heartburn (also known as GERD, or gastroesophageal reflux disease), gastritis (inflammation of the stomach lining), ulcers, and irritable bowel syndrome (IBS).

Frequent alcohol use damages the delicate linings of the GI tract and increases the risk of mouth and esophageal cancers, especially if you smoke. In fact, alcohol has been labeled a "co-carcinogen" because it works together with tobacco to significantly increase the risk of certain cancers. According to a 2006 leaflet distributed by the American Cancer Society, approximately 75 to 80 percent of all patients with oral cancer regularly consume alcohol. A 2007 report by the National Cancer Institute indicates that alcohol use increases the risk of having cancer in the mouth, larynx, liver, and esophagus. Data also indicate that women are more likely to develop breast cancer if they drink.

Your pancreas, the organ that produces insulin and helps your body digest food and process sugar, is very sensitive to alcohol's effects. Pancreatitis, an inflamed and painful pancreas, is one of the most common results of frequent alcohol use.

ALCOHOL, YOUR LIVER, AND CIRRHOSIS

The liver breaks down alcohol and removes it from your bloodstream at a relatively slow rate (one drink in one hour). Consequently, overloading the liver with too much alcohol on a regular basis has serious effects on how well that organ functions. Because the liver acts as the body's primary filter for other toxins, drugs, and substances, a liver badly damaged by alcohol affects every system in your body. Once the liver stops functioning, the body quickly dies.

Scientists still do not know exactly *how* alcohol damages the liver, but they know it does, and they know the damage occurs during the breaking-down process. Early signs of alcohol-related liver damage include alcoholic hepatitis, an inflammation of liver tissue that can cause nausea, vomiting, and fatigue. A fatty liver is another early sign of liver damage. Normally, the liver breaks down fat to produce energy for the body, but if the liver is overtaxed with breaking down alcohol, it burns the alcohol as energy instead and allows fat to build up in the liver.

Mild liver damage can be reversed—if you stop drinking—because the liver has the remarkable ability to regenerate itself. However, if frequent drinking continues, the overworked liver develops a network of scar tissue. This is called cirrhosis of the liver, and it is irreversible. Unless you have a liver transplant, cirrhosis leads to complete liver failure and premature death.

Q & A

Question: Is it possible to drown in your own vomit?

Answer: Usually, when you drink too much too quickly, a valve in your stomach begins to contract rapidly and you vomit—often more than once! This is your body's way of protecting itself from alcohol's **toxic** (poisonous) effects. If you really overdo it, however, this protective mechanism may stop working properly. If you then pass out or fall asleep and your body later tries to eliminate the alcohol as vomit, the vomit may back up into your lungs and "drown" you. Although this does not happen frequently, it is not rare. The medical term for the condition is diffuse pulmonary edema.

ALCOHOL, YOUR HEART, AND YOUR BLOOD

Frequent alcohol use raises blood pressure and heart rate, both of which make the heart work much harder to pump blood through the body. Higher blood pressure can cause a variety of problems and often needs to be controlled with medication.

Another, less common effect of frequent alcohol use is a condition called alcoholic cardiomyopathy, or "beer drinker's heart." In this disease, caused by years of excessive alcohol consumption, the heart muscle is inflamed and weakened. In advanced cases, the heart can no longer pump blood.

The major components of blood are red blood cells and white blood cells. They, too, are vulnerable to the damaging effects of alcohol. Red blood cells carry oxygen and hemoglobin, which contains iron, to all parts of the body and remove waste materials during circulation. When red blood cells are damaged by alcohol, they become sticky and cling together. This slows the blood's circulation, deprives organs and tissues of vital oxygen, and encourages blood clotting.

White blood cells are the great infection fighters and the key defensive players in your body's immune system. Some white blood cells produce antibodies that destroy infecting bacteria and viruses; others attack and kill infections directly (these are called "killer white cells"). White blood cells, which have a short life, are constantly reproducing themselves to fight infection. Alcohol damages white blood cells in three ways: it reduces the ability of the cells to create antibodies to fight infections, it impairs the process of blood cell reproduction, and it slows down the infection-fighting action of killer white cells. Damaged white blood cells make for a weak immune system.

Alcohol also damages the immune system by keeping the body from absorbing enough vitamins, minerals, and other nutrients from food. Even if you have a good, varied diet, alcohol may keep you from enjoying the full health benefits of that diet.

THE MALE REPRODUCTIVE SYSTEM

The HPG axis, or "hypothalamic-pituitary-gonadal" axis, represents the three key glands in the male reproductive system: the hypothalamus, the pituitary gland, and the gonads (or testicles). Frequent alcohol use damages all three glands and the hormones they produce. The results of this damage can include a lower sperm count and abnormal sperm, impotence (the inability to maintain an erection), shrunken testicles, and enlarged breasts. So forget about the myth that alcohol enhances sex!

JUST FOR WOMEN

Researchers are beginning to acknowledge that women are a unique group when it comes to drinking and the damaging effects of alcohol. For one thing, women are more vulnerable to alcohol-related health diseases than men. They develop liver and brain damage more quickly than men do—even when drinking *less* alcohol. In young women, frequent drinking also may interfere with bone growth or encourage bone loss, increasing the risk of osteoporosis, a bone disorder that causes bones to become porous and brittle.

As far as a young woman's reproductive system goes, excessive alcohol use inhibits the growth of the ovaries and the production of hormones that regulate ovulation, menstruation, and fertility. Frequent drinkers may have fertility problems later in life and suffer an increased rate of miscarriages. Drinking during pregnancy also can have profoundly damaging effects on the fetus.

ALCOHOL AND YOUR BRAIN

Perhaps nowhere else are the toxic effects of too much alcohol seen so quickly and dramatically as they are when alcohol hits the brain. Drinking can change your personality, lower your inhibitions, and encourage inappropriate, silly, or downright dangerous behavior.

Frequent alcohol use can change your brain's chemistry, erase parts of your memory, affect your ability to learn new tasks and make decisions, and lower your IQ. Two of the most disturbing alcohol-related brain problems are blackouts and alcohol psychosis.

Blackouts

A blackout is an alcohol-induced period of amnesia, or memory loss. It is not the same as "passing out," when you are unconscious. In a blackout, which can last seconds, minutes, or hours (or in the case of serious alcoholics, days or weeks), a person appears normal (though usually drunk) to the outside world, as he or she talks and interacts with others. But he or she later has no memory of that time. The person cannot remember what was said or done, or who he or she was with, and will never be able to retrieve that memory, not even under hypnosis. This is called an "en bloc blackout," or total blackout, and is the most common form of blacking out. Sometimes, people have what are called "fragmentary blackouts," where partial memory is restored when something jogs the recollection.

Scientists used to believe that only serious alcoholics had blackouts, but now experts agree that even one episode of overdrinking can cause a blackout.

It is a frightening phenomenon to the drinker, but in the best-case scenario, he or she is probably just embarrassed. At the worst-case end of the spectrum, what happens during a blackout can change one's life forever.

TEENS SPEAK

He Can't Remember a Thing

"It was so scary. You don't know what it's like until it happens to you." That's how one seventeen-year-old alcoholic describes the times he blacked out while drinking.

Now Carey goes to Alcoholics Anonymous meetings twice a week; he had been sober for a few months when he told his story. But Carey is the first to admit that he might never have done anything about his problem if he hadn't started to get blackouts.

"I used to brag about how I could hold my liquor. I was getting better and better at it; I even made money a couple of times by betting I could drink older guys under the table. My father is a heavy drinker and my uncle too, but they're not alcoholics, really; I never saw my dad drive drunk, or go to work drunk or anything like that. So I had their examples to aspire to.

"First it was beer, then vodka. By then I was drinking so much on the weekends, I had to steal money from my mother's pocketbook just to pay for the liquor. At the beginning, I felt like I was in control. After a while, I would get really drunk every time I drank. Like the vodka was finally getting to me. I wasn't a happy drunk; I was confused and upset that I wasn't in control anymore. Then I'd find myself waking up on some couch, and I couldn't remember how I got there.

"It was like some kind of time or space warp. The last thing I would remember was getting together with my friends to drink, but what happened later? I would try and try to remember, but it didn't come back. I thought I was losing my mind.

"After that, I was scared enough to talk to my minister at church about it. He put me in touch with A.A.."

Alcohol psychosis

Alcohol **psychosis** is a group of brain-related symptoms that occur after frequent, heavy drinking, often during alcohol **withdrawal**, the combination of painful and uncomfortable symptoms alcoholics feel when they stop or drastically cut back their drinking. The symptoms are similar to those of the psychiatric disorder called *schizophrenia* and can include auditory and visual **hallucinations** (seeing and hearing things that aren't there); convulsions (violent shaking of the body); delusions; phobias, which are excessive and persistent fears; violent language and/or behavior; and **delirium tremens** (commonly called "the D.T.'s"), which are intense, terrifying mental images that can happen if a person stops drinking for three to four days and are accompanied by high fevers and extremely aggressive behavior. The D.T.'s involve profound anxiety and insomnia along with convulsions. Alcohol psychosis is a serious, life-threatening condition that requires hospitalization.

WHAT YOU DON'T KNOW WILL HARM YOU

Considering alcohol's role in human diseases, smart people handle it with caution and care. However, the results show that millions of people do not follow that good example. Fortunately, you are at an age where you can make wise choices that can help you live a long and happy life.

See also: Alcohol and Violence; Binge Drinking Among Teenagers; Birth Defects and Alcohol; Effects on the Body; Sexual Behavior and Alcohol; Withdrawal

FURTHER READING

Steward, Gail. *Fetal Alcohol Syndrome.* Diseases and Disorders. Chicago: Lucent Books, 2004.

Volkmann, Chris, and Toren Volkmann. *From Binge to Blackout: A Mother and Son Struggle with Teen Drinking.* New American Library, New York: 2006.

Watson, Ronald, and Adam K. Meyers, eds. *Alcohol and Heart Disease.* New York: Taylor and Francis, 2002.

■ ALCOHOL AND VIOLENCE

For the majority of people who drink, alcohol is a way to relax, to help them socialize with friends, and to put aside the pressures and tensions of life. But from time immemorial, alcohol has been associated with arguments, fights, brawls, rape, spousal and child abuse,

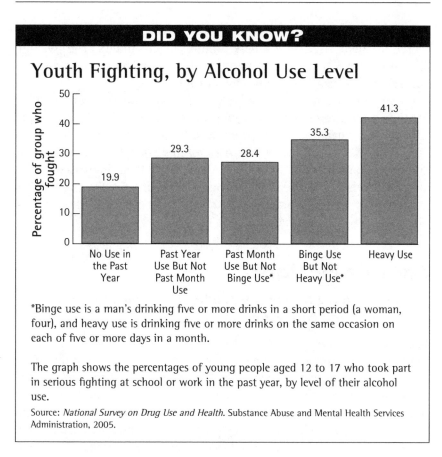

DID YOU KNOW?

Youth Fighting, by Alcohol Use Level

Percentage of group who fought

No Use in the Past Year	19.9
Past Year Use But Not Past Month Use	29.3
Past Month Use But Not Binge Use*	28.4
Binge Use But Not Heavy Use*	35.3
Heavy Use	41.3

*Binge use is a man's drinking five or more drinks in a short period (a woman, four), and heavy use is drinking five or more drinks on the same occasion on each of five or more days in a month.

The graph shows the percentages of young people aged 12 to 17 who took part in serious fighting at school or work in the past year, by level of their alcohol use.

Source: *National Survey on Drug Use and Health.* Substance Abuse and Mental Health Services Administration, 2005.

and even suicide. In the often-quoted words of the 1993 "Special Report to the U.S. Congress on Alcohol and Health," the secretary of health and human services wrote, "Alcohol is associated with a substantial proportion of human violence, and perpetrators [those who commit crimes] are often under the influence of alcohol."

How can one substance have such contradictory effects? And what can individuals do to make sure that they are never the perpetrator or the victim of a violent alcohol-related act?

HOSTILITY AND AGGRESSION

Violence, when one person physically harms or tries to harm another person, is the most severe form of the more general behavior called *aggression*. Aggression also can be conveyed through words—hostile remarks, insults, threats, and hurtful gossip. A person can hurt other people emotionally, or harm them by spreading lies or betraying secrets to their friends, teachers, family, or coworkers. The average person may never witness criminal violence, but he or she probably will see and hear a loud, obnoxious drunk.

To the victim, any form of aggression can be frightening. If it continues on a regular basis, it can make the victim's life miserable. Alcohol has been shown to promote aggression in all its forms. In fact, a study reported in 2000 in *Alcohol and Alcoholism* showed that aggression among men increased along with their increased blood alcohol levels (until the level got high enough to make the drinker unable to act at all). Women in this study, as in others in the past, did not show the same correlation.

Fact Or Fiction?

Cheap hard liquor is more likely to lead to violence than fine wine.

The Facts: Nonsense! A glass of wine and a shot of liquor have exactly the same effect on anyone. True, a group of close friends sipping wine and sampling cheese in a neighborhood pub, with soothing music in the background, will probably not get into a fight over a misunderstood remark. But they would be just as cool and relaxed if they were sipping bourbon or scotch. On the other hand, a tired, angry loner sitting in a noisy bar ordering one drink after another may be at risk of violence, whether he is drinking the finest European wine or the cheapest whiskey on the market.

In most cases of alcohol-related aggression and violence, one cannot put all the blame on alcohol. Very few people in happy marriages assault their spouses, even under the influence of alcohol. A law-abiding, stable citizen does not suddenly knock down and rob a passerby every time he's had "a few too many."

People who have a history of violent behavior, or who tend to be aggressive even without alcohol, may be more vulnerable to the violence-provoking effects of alcohol. Still, the statistical connection between alcohol and different forms of violence is strong enough to suggest that something about alcohol itself brings out the worst in many individuals.

WHAT IS THE MECHANISM?

Psychologists have come up with a couple of basic theories about how alcohol contributes to aggression. The most popular theory is the **disinhibition model.** This theory says that alcohol chemically blurs or deadens the parts of the brain that inhibit, or hold back, one's first impulsive reactions. In nonscientific words, when you're drunk, you lose control.

When people feel insulted or threatened, or think that someone is treating them unfairly, their first impulse may be to lash out in retaliation. But normally they control that impulse. Their better judgment tells them that a) they may have misunderstood or misinterpreted the other person, and b) it probably isn't worth fighting about, and c) in any case, if they fight, they might get hurt.

Any time two people strongly disagree, the disagreement has the potential to become nasty, or even violent. Fighting is usually the "easy" way out. It is harder and more challenging to find a delicate compromise, to think of a less offensive way of making a point or to simply "agree to disagree." Unfortunately, alcohol makes that even harder to achieve, by numbing a drinker's mental faculties.

If this theory is true, anyone has the potential to become aggressive under the influence of alcohol when faced with provocation or threats. But the people most at risk are those who are prone to violence even when sober.

Some researchers have recently tried to figure out the precise mechanism behind disinhibition. For example, according to psychologist James W. Kalat, in the 2001 book *Biological Psychology,* alcohol may reduce the activity of serotonin, a chemical messenger in the brain that is believed to act as an inhibitor. Other key brain chemicals involved in behavior and mood, such as dopamine, may also be disrupted by alcohol.

The second theory is called **alcohol expectancy.** This theory claims that in some cultures, people believe that alcohol all by itself can turn a drinker violent. When people with that notion drink, they almost expect to get into fights. In some laboratory studies, people became more aggressive after drinking a nonalcoholic beverage that they *believed* was alcohol. Similarly, some criminals say they use alcohol to overcome their fears and inhibitions before committing a violent crime. They too believe in the equation: Alcohol means aggression. These expectations may encourage the behavior.

These theories are interesting, but they may not tell the full story. Sometimes, an emotional problem makes people act in a hostile and aggressive manner, *and* the same problem leads them to abuse alcohol as an escape. In those cases, it is not accurate to say that alcohol abuse caused the violence; they are both the result of the *underlying* emotional cause.

There may be another reason to take the statistics about alcohol and crime with a grain of salt. Common sense tells us that criminals under the influence of alcohol may not be careful about hiding their tracks; that probably makes it easier for the police to find them. Because sober criminals may be more likely to escape detection, they do not wind up in the statistics. In other words, it may *look* as if all the perpetrators are drinking, because the ones who don't drink are not caught.

There is also a feedback effect between violence and alcohol. People who have been victimized by violence are more likely to abuse alcohol; under the influence, they may in turn commit violence against other people. This can happen within families, as each new generation repeats the patterns learned from the previous one.

VIOLENT CRIMES

In a 1997 report, the National Institute on Alcohol Abuse and Alcoholism reported that a very high percentage of murderers were drinking at the time of their crimes—as many as 86 percent of them in some areas. Up to 37 percent of those committing assault also had been drinking. Most other categories of crime showed similar high correlations with alcohol, including sexual assault and rape. According to the Bureau of Justice Statistics, between 2001 and 2005, victims reported that alcohol or drugs were in use in approximately 42 percent of nonfatal cases of domestic violence.

Robbery also gets into the picture. Robbers need a clear head to plan and carry out their crimes, yet, according to a 2001 article in *Alcohol Research and Health*, nearly one third of the people jailed for robbery say they had been drinking at the time of the crime. The article also reported that a 1998 survey of violent offenders found that 38 percent of those in state prisons, 41 percent of those in local jails, and 41 percent of those on probation "reported that they had been using alcohol when they committed their offenses."

You may be saying to yourself, "This is not *me*. I would never attack another person, no matter how much alcohol I drink." That may be true, yet the issue may still affect you more than you think, because a large percentage of the *victims* of violent crimes were also drinking when the crimes were committed.

Without intending to, people can sometimes innocently provoke a violent attack. The recipe for violence often is: violent tendencies (on the part of the aggressor), too much alcohol, and a word or gesture (by the victim) that is misinterpreted as a provocation.

People under the influence of alcohol are not likely to be tactful. They may say or do things, with no malicious intent, that they would never say or do when sober. As they continue to dig themselves into a hole, they may be too drunk to notice the facial expressions and body language of others that should be flashing the warning: "Change the subject, sit down, stop waving your arms in the air." None of this excuses the person who commits a violent act, but it does suggest that being even mildly intoxicated can sometimes be quite dangerous even for a nonviolent individual.

Finally, when you are drunk, you are an easy target for criminals. For example, you may exercise poor judgment while alone in an isolated area. And when danger approaches, you may not be able to talk your way out of it or, if need be, to run away.

SEXUAL ASSAULT AND RAPE

Every major study on the subject of rape and sexual assault shows a strong correlation between these crimes and alcohol. Very often, both the perpetrator and the victim had been drinking when the crime took place.

Apart from the general link between alcohol and violence, additional factors are involved in sexual crimes. The male perpetrator may believe that alcohol enhances his sexual abilities. In fact, studies have shown that it does the opposite; it is generally harder for a man to perform sexually after drinking more than a minimum amount.

The perpetrator may also believe in some old-fashioned myths about women and alcohol, which sensible people have long ago discarded. For example, he may believe that "nice" women do not drink in public, so any woman who does so is probably available for sex. He may assume that a woman who agrees to drink with him is giving him license to take sexual advantage of her. Or he may honestly misinterpret her words and behavior—alcohol can prevent people from "reading" the complicated clues and hidden messages that govern sexual behavior.

Rapists often "excuse" their behavior by blaming alcohol, and they may even drink in advance in order to give themselves an excuse.

They also may knowingly exploit the fact that women get intoxicated on smaller amounts of alcohol and deliberately get women to drink too much.

The female victim may also allow alcohol to cloud her judgment. Most women become intoxicated much sooner after drinking the same amount of alcohol as a man. Their ability to communicate their desires, including the decision not to engage in sexual behavior, may be impaired. And when the attack begins, women may not have all the mental and physical resources they need to fend it off.

CHILD ABUSE

Some of the saddest cases of alcohol-related violence involve child abuse. This can include incest, usually committed by fathers, or physical abuse, which mothers are as likely to commit as fathers.

The National Center on Addiction and Substance Abuse at Columbia University issued some frightening figures in a 1999 report. Children whose parents abuse alcohol and other drugs are 2.7 times more likely to physically abuse their children. Most child welfare and court professionals told the researchers that alcohol and other drugs caused, or contributed to, more than half of all cases of physical abuse. It should be noted, however, that scientific surveys of the evidence do not always show that alcohol is the cause of violent child abuse.

When a parent is drunk, any kind of normal childhood behavior can trigger a violent response. Older kids may learn to avoid their parents or to withdraw emotionally. Younger kids, however, may simply be unable to keep themselves from crying, disobeying, or somehow annoying their parents.

Alcohol is estimated to be involved in close to half of all reported cases of incest. In addition, even parents who do not themselves abuse their children may, if they abuse alcohol, be unable to prevent other adults, sometimes alcohol abusers themselves, from harming their children.

TEENS SPEAK

I Still Cry When I Remember

Seth's mother is now in recovery, and they get along fine when she comes to visit. But he still gets very emotional when he lets himself think of the period last year when she really cracked.

"It's not like we didn't know she was an alcoholic. I was thirteen years old then, but even my younger brother Jordan understood that Mom had a problem with booze. When she would drink, in the afternoons before Dad came home, we used to steer clear. Any little thing would tick her off and she'd start yelling and hitting us—not hard, just to get us away from her. But she would always come in to apologize before we went to bed.

"Then Mom and Dad started to fight. He used to drink a little too, and he'd call her names, like say she was a lousy mother and things. She'd scream at him, and sometimes they threw punches. Then he would leave and slam the door.

"Then one time last year, she took a real swing at Jordan, and he fell against the edge of the table. He started screaming, and I saw he had a big gash right under his eye. Mom told me to call 911, but she was too drunk to come with the ambulance; they had to call Dad.

"In the end Jordan had three stitches; he'll probably always have this big scar.

"I was so mad at Mom at first, but when we came home she fell all over us crying, and apologized a million times. It was really pathetic; I just hated her and wouldn't let her off the hook. But now I understand better; it was really the liquor talking, not Mom. Since she went sober we get along much better."

SPOUSAL ABUSE

Of all violent crimes, spousal abuse is the one most associated with alcohol. The authors of a 2005 article in the *Journal of Consulting and Clinical Psychology* found that heavy drinking was related to committing serious violent acts. Individuals who drank heavily were four times more likely to commit serious violence against partners on that day compared to days where they were not drinking heavily. Also, authors of a 2006 study in *Alcoholism: Clinical and Experimental Research* discovered similar findings. White soldiers were almost four times more likely to engage in domestic violence if they had between eight and 14 drinks a week. African-American soldiers were almost three times more likely to engage in domestic violence if they also had between eight and 14 drinks per week.

Broader studies show that between 60 and 70 percent of spousal violence cases involve alcohol. Usually, both partners have been drinking. Clearly, these incidents involve many other issues apart from just alcohol. Sometimes, when alcohol abuse itself is a major subject of contention between the partners, one partner taking a single drink can trigger a violent confrontation.

Cultural approval of violence is the strongest factor that determines whether or not an argument between spouses or partners may escalate to violence. In other words, if a man believes that his religion, ethnic group, or community grants him a right to dominate his partner or to use force, he may well act on that belief. On the other hand, if he believes spousal abuse will be met with disapproval in his social circles, he is less likely to use that type of force.

In many cases of spousal violence, the female partner is involved in violent behavior as well as the male, and she may have had as much to drink. However, women are more likely than men to suffer moderate or severe physical violence and harm, even in cases where they initiated the violence.

SELF-MUTILATION

Self-mutilation, or deliberate self-harm, is a serious emotional disorder that affects many teenagers, more often girls than boys. It may include hitting, cutting or burning one's skin, pulling one's hair, and even taking poison. The individual does not want to do any lasting harm, but he or she cannot control the impulse. No one knows why some kids behave this way, but some therapists believe they are trying to cover up emotional pain with physical pain.

Kids who mutilate themselves also may abuse alcohol or other drugs. In some cases, alcohol or drug use can worsen the problem by contributing to feelings of low self-esteem and hopelessness.

SUICIDE

About 33,000 Americans kill themselves every year, and many thousands more attempt suicide. The American Foundation for Suicide Prevention currently reports that alcoholism is a factor in approximately 30 percent of completed suicides. Also, a 2009 report by the CDC indicates that approximately 24 percent of those who committed suicide had a blood alcohol level of .08 or higher. Even worse, alcohol is particularly associated with unplanned, impulsive suicides rather than with premeditated acts. Because alcohol can reduce inhibitions, impair judgment, and make depression worse, any one of those effects could push a suicidal person over the edge.

According to the American Foundation for Suicide Prevention, in 2005 approximately 30 percent of all completed suicides involved alcohol. Also, in a leaflet distributed by the CDC in 2008, researchers reported that 33.3 percent of suicide victims tested positive for alcohol. (The figure rises to three times as likely for kids who use illegal drugs, apart from marijuana.)

The lesson is clear. Anyone unhappy enough to have considered ending his or her life must be very careful about choosing whether, where, when, and with whom to drink.

Q & A

Question: How common is suicide among young people? Isn't it really an adult problem?

Answer: Unfortunately, suicide is common among adolescents in the United States. It is the fourth leading cause of death for kids aged 10 to 14 and the third leading cause of death in the 15 to 25 age group. If you are depressed about your problems and feel like ending it all, why not give yourself another chance? Instead of picking up a bottle, pick up the phone and get help—from a friend, relative, teacher, doctor, or hot line.

A COMMON PROBLEM

Whatever the cause-and-effect relationship may be, alcohol is associated with violence of many different kinds. Anyone who drinks, or plans to drink, should keep this relationship in mind. If an individual, a particular situation, or a setting has the potential for violence, sensible people will stay away from that next drink—or any drink at all.

See also: Alcohol and Depression; Drinking on College Campuses; Sexual Behavior and Alcohol

FURTHER READING
Dingwall, Gavin. *Alcohol and Crime.* Devon, U.K.: Willan Publishing, 2006.
Farrington, David P., and Brandon C. Welsch. *Saving Children from a Life of Crime: Early Risk Factors and Effective Interventions.* New York: Oxford University Press, 2008.

Greenfield, Lawrence A. *Alcohol and Crime: An Analysis of National Data on the Prevalence of Alcohol Involvement in Crime.* Washington, D.C.: Bureau of Justice Statistics, 1998.

Parker, Robert Nash. *Alcohol and Crime: A Deadly Combination of Two American Traditions.* Albany: State University of New York Press, 1995.

■ ALCOHOLISM, CAUSES OF

Despite decades of research and the efforts of many scientists, no one has discovered a single, definitive cause of alcoholism, also known as the addiction to alcohol, or the physical and emotional dependency on alcohol. In fact, so many theories about alcoholism have evolved over the last two centuries that when noted alcohol scholar E.-M. Jellinek wrote his famous 1960 book *The Disease Concept of Alcoholism,* he identified more than 200 theories and definitions of alcoholism.

Historical theories of alcoholism include the moral and temperance models of the 19th and early 20th centuries. In the 1930s, the "alcoholism as a disease" concept became popular and is still the prevailing theory in many recovery movements. Less popular, but equally important, are theories that attempt to factor in the unique personality, social, cultural, or behavioral characteristics of alcoholics.

Starting in the 1970s, scientists who had long suspected a biological cause of alcohol abuse began studying **alcoholics** for genetic (physical traits inherited from parents) and biochemical similarities. By the end of the 20th century, researchers had indeed found a strong biological component to alcoholism.

Nevertheless, all experts agree that social, cultural, and emotional factors play a major role in alcohol abuse as well. For example, kids who grow up in communities or social groups where getting drunk is acceptable may eventually become alcoholics, even if none of them seem to have biological tendencies in that direction. In other words, alcoholism has multiple causes.

Here is a brief look at some of the more popular theories about the cause of alcoholism.

THE MORALITY AND TEMPERANCE THEORIES

The **morality theory** of alcoholism places the blame squarely on the individual. Put simply, the theory proposes that responsible people with strong moral fiber do not drink; weak-willed people with no spiritual backbone *do* drink–in fact, they drink too much and get in a lot of trouble. This was a popular theory in the 18th and 19th centuries. While it sounds puritanical and old-fashioned, the idea that alcoholics are deviant people with no willpower is one that still persists in many people's views today.

The **temperance movement** that began in the late 18th century and thrived in the 19th had its own theory of alcoholism. It shifted the blame for alcohol abuse from the individual to alcohol itself. While at first the movement favored moderate drinking, over time it began to view alcohol as an inherently dangerous substance that no one could drink safely in any amount.

The temperance movement in the United States culminated in 1919 in the passage of the Eighteenth Amendment to the U.S. Constitution, which prohibited the manufacture and sale of alcohol. **Prohibition** (which *prohibited* the sale of alcoholic beverages), lasted for 14 years. Though the law did indeed cause a major reduction in drinking and alcohol abuse, especially outside urban areas, it also generated some major problems of its own. For example, organized crime flourished, as there was still a demand for alcohol. Those gangs who engaged in bootlegging–the making, selling, or transporting alcohol–had plenty of opportunities to profit. According to the Digital History Web site, the infamous Chicago gangster Al Capone's group took in an estimated $60 million in 1927 alone. Public opinion turned against Prohibition, and in 1933 the Twenty-first Amendment put an end to the experiment.

THE DISEASE THEORY

Two years after Prohibition ended in 1933, the **Alcoholics Anonymous** (A.A.) program began, and A.A. groups sprang up across the United States. Proponents of the A.A. program of recovery claimed that alcoholism was a progressive, incurable, and potentially fatal disease to which a certain small group of individuals–alcoholics–were uniquely susceptible. According to the **disease theory,** alcoholics (who can never drink safely) are physically different from nonalcoholics (who can drink safely). Since alcoholism has no cure, the **recovering alcoholic** must practice lifelong sobriety: He or she must never drink again.

The disease theory of alcoholism was embraced strongly by alcoholics and nonalcoholics alike, as well as by the liquor industry and the medical community. Today, it is still a powerful concept in recovery programs and among physicians and substance abuse counselors.

Though a small but vocal group believe that alcoholics can learn to drink moderately and safely, most experts encourage alcohol abusers to give up drinking entirely.

THE PERSONALITY, SOCIOCULTURAL, AND BEHAVIORAL THEORIES

Personality theories of alcoholism have their roots in psychoanalysis, a method of investigating mental processes by means of confronting repressed thoughts. In the 1940s and 1950s, psychiatrists proposed several theories about alcoholics. One suggested that alcoholics had never progressed beyond some critical stage in their personality development, usually the "oral stage," the primary focus of the first months of a baby's life when pleasure derives from things in the mouth. Other theories considered alcoholics to have low self-esteem or to suffer from sex-role or sexual identity conflicts. These theories are not widely accepted today.

Psychologists, social workers, and substance abuse counselors have long identified various social and cultural causes of alcohol abuse. They believe that people who belong to social circles where heavy drinking is the norm (such as various professions or ethnic groups), or who live in places where alcohol is available and cheap or in subcultures that associate alcohol with drunkenness, are more likely to abuse the beverage, whatever their underlying personalities. They also believe people can become dependent on alcohol due to financial or emotional stress, poor coping skills, and susceptibility to peer pressure.

The behavioral theory considers alcoholism to be a learned behavior. **Conditioning** by the family and the community, reinforced by peers and even by liquor advertising, can teach people unhealthy behavior patterns, to the extent that the first drink, or even the sight of a bar on a street, kicks off a chain of events leading to intoxication. Treatment usually involves **counterconditioning,** or behavioral therapy, in which the alcoholic learns new, healthier ways of responding to the stimulus of alcohol.

Fact Or Fiction?

Three million American teens are alcoholics.

The Facts: Yes. The National Institute of Alcoholism and Alcohol Abuse reported in 2000 that nearly 3 million young people between the ages of

14 and 17 "are regular drinkers with a serious alcohol problem," a figure that still stands today. Typically, their first experience of alcohol intoxication occurs in the early to mid-teens. Historically, teenage boys drank more alcohol than teenage girls, but in recent years the gap between the genders has almost disappeared.

BIOLOGICAL THEORIES:
HEREDITY, GENETICS, AND BIOCHEMISTRY

For centuries, medical experts and lay people alike have observed that alcohol abuse runs in families and seems to be passed down from one generation to the next. That fact has become a given. The real question is: Why? The challenge to researchers is figuring out how to separate "nature from nurture" in the development of family-related alcoholism. In other words, are children of alcoholics at a higher risk for alcoholism because they inherited a gene that makes it difficult to handle alcohol ("nature"), or do they learn alcoholic behaviors from observing their parents as they grow up ("nurture")?

In recent decades, scientists have tried to discover a possible genetic link to alcoholism by looking at twins and at children adopted into or out of alcoholic families.

Heredity: twin and adoption studies

Studies of twins and of adoptions have served to highlight the role genetics play in alcohol use and abuse. Identical (or monozygotic) twins share the same genes. Fraternal (or dizygotic) twins share no more genes than other brothers and sisters. The authors of an article that was published in a 2009 edition of *Addiction* review evidence of the role both genes and environment have on alcohol use. The evidence shows that beyond all doubt, there is a genetic component to alcohol use, abuse, and addiction. Identical twins are more likely to both abuse alcohol than fraternal twins.

Adoption studies also provide evidence that genes are involved in alcohol use and abuse. In 2008, in a study published in *Addiction*, the authors reported having reviewed evidence provided by studies of adoptions. Children whose biological parents were alcoholics are significantly more likely to abuse alcohol, even though they are raised by another family. In fact, the environment of the adoptive family plays a weaker role in alcohol abuse than the genetic connection between the biological parent and the child. Another 2009 study in *Addiction* reported on the influence of genetics versus environment for alcohol use and abuse. The authors of this study also found that genes play a significant role in this problem. Approximately 32 percent of adopted children who admitted to using alcohol had been exposed to alcohol problems by at least one parent. Only 8.3 percent of adopted children who admitted to using alcohol had not been exposed to alcohol problems by a parent. However, 41.3 percent of biological children admitted to using alcohol, even though they had not been exposed to alcohol problems by a parent. Amazingly, there were almost eight times as many biological children who used alcohol when compared to adopted children, even though neither of these groups had witnessed problems with alcohol by their parents!

Q & A

Question: My big sister was lecturing me about not drinking. She says that since my parents are alcoholics and because I'm a boy, I could become an alcoholic too. Is that true?

Answer: Between 20 and 25 percent of the sons and brothers of alcoholics become alcoholics themselves. In contrast, only 5 percent of the daughters and sisters of alcoholics become alcoholics. However, whether male or female, child or sibling, those with a genetic tendency for alcoholism are more likely to begin abusing alcohol at a younger age than their peers, become alcoholic sooner, and have a more severe form of alcoholism. More reasons, if you come from a family with a history of alcohol abuse, to think long and hard before picking up that first drink.

Genetics and biochemistry
In the 1990s, the National Institute of Alcohol Abuse and Alcoholism (NIAAA) and the Collaborative Study on the Genetics of Alcoholism (COGA) launched a long-term study to identify the actual genes that may cause alcoholism. Researchers are analyzing the genetic makeup of 1,000 individuals from families with a history of alcoholism. To date, scientists have identified a possible strong genetic link to increased alcohol **dependence** on chromosomes 1 and 7, and a more modest link for dependence on chromosome 2.

Researchers have also identified genetic variations that may work to *prevent* alcoholism. These variations are in the genes that produce enzymes that speed up the body's metabolism, or breaking down process, of alcohol. When the body breaks down alcohol quickly, a large amount of the toxic chemical **acetaldehyde** is released, making the drinker feel sick and "flushed." In general, people who suffer this reaction avoid alcohol, or drink very little. For example, there is a relatively low rate of alcoholism among East Asians, many of whom have the genes that cause them to experience the flushing reaction when they drink even a small amount of alcohol (as reported by the NIAAA in 1998). The unpleasant sensations more than balance out the "high" they may get from alcohol.

The NIAAA and COGA researchers found that individuals from alcoholic families who did *not* become alcohol abusers themselves had these protective genes. These people appear to have a built-in genetic protection against abusing alcohol.

Acetaldehyde also figures prominently in some studies linking brain chemistry and alcoholism. For instance, acetaldehyde combines with other chemicals in the brain to produce compounds called TIQs. TIQs chemically resemble morphine, a powerfully addictive opiate. This process may account for the "craving" for alcohol that many alcohol abusers experience.

Thus, a single by-product of alcohol can have opposite effects on different people. For those who break down alcohol quickly, high levels of acetaldehyde produce unpleasant symptoms that turn them off alcohol. For those who break down alcohol gradually, the same chemical helps create powerful cravings for the beverage.

Alcohol also appears to increase or decrease levels of certain brain chemicals, notably serotonin, a complex chemical in the brain that transmits nerve signals. An imbalance in serotonin levels has been linked to depression; when levels are restored, a feeling of well-being seems to result. To the extent that alcohol may increase serotonin levels, some drinkers may be unwittingly "medicating themselves" when they drink.

Some alcoholics show imbalances in brain chemistry, according to George F. Koob, head of an NIAAA research program on the microbiology of alcoholism. Koob said in April 2003 that some alcoholics may have a hyperactive stress system, and may be using alcohol just "to feel normal." However it is not clear whether the imbalance causes alcoholism or vice versa.

GENETICS—AND EVERYTHING ELSE

Most experts now agree that genetics plays a major role in the development of alcoholism. They generally estimate that between 40 and

60 percent of the risk for alcoholism is genetic. But genetics is not the only cause. Ongoing research should clarify the relative role of the other factors, including social and psychological problems and the influence of subcultures and peer groups.

See also: Alcohol Abuse, the Risks of; Alcohol and Depression; Alcohol and Violence; Alcohol, History of; Drinking and Drugs; Recovery and Treatment; Underage Drinking

FURTHER READING

Asbury, William F., and Katherine Ketcham. *Beyond the Influence: Understanding and Defeating Alcoholism.* New York: Bantam Books, 2000.

Herrick, Charles. *100 Q&A About Alcoholism & Drug Addiction.* Sudbury, Mass.: Jones and Bartlett Publishers, 2007.

Lawson, Ann W., and Gary Lawson. *Alcoholism and the Family: A Guide to Treatment and Prevention.* Austin, Tex.: Pro-Ed Publishers, 2004.

Marshall, Ronald. *Alcoholism: Genetic Culpability or Social Irresponsibility.* Lanham, Md: University Press of America, 2001.

ALCOHOL POISONING

Body's reaction to **toxic** levels of alcohol in the blood. Alcohol is a poison. By drinking any amount of alcohol, a person is allowing a poison to enter the body. However, when we talk about alcohol poisoning, we refer to the consequences of drinking too much alcohol in a short period of time. Binge drinking, which means drinking five or more drinks (four or more for women) within a short period of time, is the primary cause of alcohol poisoning.

Drinking too much alcohol overloads the body; it cannot effectively process and eliminate the poison. Further, alcohol is a **depressant,** and too much can cause the body to shut down. As a result, alcohol poisoning can be fatal.

CAUSES AND SYMPTOMS OF ALCOHOL POISONING

Binge drinking is the main cause of alcohol poisoning. Binge drinking is defined as rapidly drinking five or more drinks in less than two

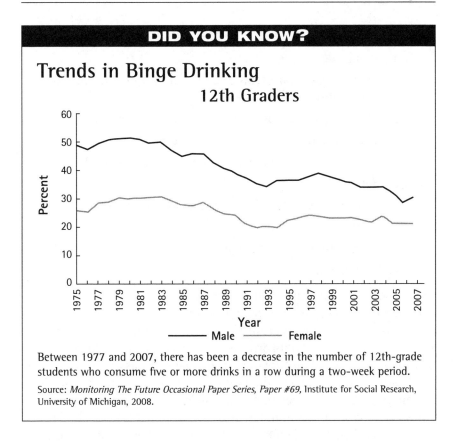

Trends in Binge Drinking
12th Graders

Between 1977 and 2007, there has been a decrease in the number of 12th-grade students who consume five or more drinks in a row during a two-week period.

Source: *Monitoring The Future Occasional Paper Series, Paper #69,* Institute for Social Research, University of Michigan, 2008.

hours. Women are binge drinking if they consume four or more drinks in two hours. The National Institute of Alcohol Abuse and Alcoholism states that binge drinking is a pattern of drinking that will bring a person's **blood alcohol content** to .08 or higher. For example, quickly drinking one beer, then another and another, is binge drinking. The body does not have sufficient time to **metabolize,** or break down, all the alcohol in its system.

People vary as to how well they metabolize alcohol. Alcohol cannot be stored in the body; it must be processed. Metabolization occurs in both the stomach and the liver, although most of the process takes place in the liver.

It is important to know if a person is suffering from alcohol poisoning. Because people can die from this, the sooner one receives medical treatment, the better.

Symptoms to look for include the following:

1. Vomiting
2. Slow or irregular breathing, FEWER than eight breaths per minute
3. Vomiting while unconscious and not waking up
4. Low body temperature, or hypothermia
5. Unconscious or semiconscious and cannot be awakened
6. Seizures
7. Pale or bluish skin that is also cold and clammy
8. Confusion
9. No reaction to painful stimuli
10. No reflexes

Alcohol is quickly absorbed by the body. On an empty stomach, it can take less than a minute for alcohol to reach your brain. Nausea and then vomiting are typically the first symptoms associated with alcohol poisoning. Alcohol irritates the stomach—too much and the body is forced to try and remove it. If a person passes out and alcohol is still in the stomach, the body will try to absorb or expel it. It is important to remember that someone's blood alcohol content can continue to rise for 90 minutes after the person's last drink if his or her stomach is empty. Someone can pass out from drinking, and his or her blood alcohol content can continue to increase.

Q & A

Question: Is it safe to simply "sleep it off" if someone has passed out and may have alcohol poisoning?

Answer: No. Letting someone sleep it off is dangerous. If someone has passed out and is unresponsive, medical attention should be sought immediately. The body cannot function properly with alcohol in it, and too much can cause the body to shut down. A person can choke to death by vomiting while unconscious. One can also stop breathing, fall into a coma, or develop brain damage. If you suspect someone is suffering from alcohol poisoning, call 911 and let medical professionals care for the person.

Alcohol is not only a psychological depressant but also a physical one. Physically, it depresses nerves, such as those needed for breathing and for a gag reflex (which is important for vomiting). Too much alcohol will stop these bodily functions. A lethal dose of alcohol occurs when a person's blood alcohol is concentrated between .40 and .50. This concentration will lead to death for half of the population.

FATALITIES FROM ALCOHOL POISONING

Compared to other alcohol-related topics, there is not much research on alcohol poisoning. Because the effects of alcohol on the body are well known, little research is needed.

The Substance Abuse and Mental Health Services Administration, part of the U.S. Department of Health and Human Services, published a report in 2008 that examined hospital emergency department visits related to drugs and alcohol. The data come from DAWN, the Drug Abuse Warning Network. Information on alcohol-related visits are collected when one of the following conditions is met: (1) alcohol and other drugs are found in a person's body; or (2) alcohol alone is found and the person is under the age of 21. In 2008, approximately 577,521 visits to an emergency department were alcohol-related. Of these visits, 450,817 involved both alcohol and another drug. An estimated 155,708 patients had to be admitted to a hospital for care, while 26,283 were referred to a **detoxification** program.

Approximately 125,888 people under the age of 21 had to go to the emergency department for an alcohol-related problem. Of these, only 7,479 had to be admitted to the hospital, while another 1,962 were referred to a detox program.

A 2004 study in the *Journal of Studies on Alcohol* provides some insight into the prevalence of alcohol poisoning. The authors estimate that in 2000 there were 231 men and an estimated 70 women who died from alcohol poisoning. That translates to almost six deaths per week.

One of the more extensive studies on alcohol poisoning comes from the National Institute on Alcohol Abuse and Alcoholism. Using data from 1996 through 1998, the institute estimated that an average of seven deaths occurred each year from alcohol poisoning through alcoholic beverages. However, an average of 150 people died each year through alcohol poisoning by "other and unspecified ethyl alcohol and its products." In other words, there was not enough documentation to conclusively state that the alcohol poisoning was a result of drinking alcoholic beverages.

However, the study did highlight one very important finding: Accidental alcohol poisoning was a contributing factor in many other deaths. An average of 1,076 deaths per year occurred where accidental alcohol poisoning played a role. Taking other drugs while intoxicated accounted for an average of 955 deaths per year.

International data also provide some insight on alcohol poisoning. A 2003 study in the *British Medical Journal* examined mortality trends in Russia. The authors found that in 1991 an estimated 8.8 men per 100,000 died from alcohol poisoning. By 2001, this number jumped to 17.4 per 100,000. Women, on the other hand, were much less likely to die as a result of alcohol poisoning. In 1991, 0.9 women per 100,000 died from alcohol poisoning. This number climbed to 3.5 per 100,000 by 2001.

The authors of a 2002 study in the journal *Addiction* studied fatal alcohol poisoning in Finland. From 1983 to 1999, there were 6,179 fatal alcohol poisonings. Most of the victims were males, with females accounting for 1,072 deaths. The authors found that these fatalities peaked at various points during the year. The peaks occur during May Day (May 1), Midsummer Day (the Saturday closest to June 24), and Christmas. During these festive periods, parties and drinking are more popular, increasing the chances of someone getting alcohol poisoning. The authors also found that sales of spirits, as opposed to beer or wine, were directly related to fatal alcohol poisonings. As sales increased, so did fatal alcohol poisonings. This makes sense, as spirits have more alcohol by volume than beer or wine. By comparison, most beer has no more than 6 percent alcohol by volume, while wine typically does not exceed 16 percent.

Authors of a 2005 study in *Addiction* examined mortality resulting from alcohol poisoning in Poland. The authors found that men were 10 times more likely to die from alcohol poisoning than women. Those who were more educated were less likely to die from alcohol poisoning than those with less education.

According to the authors of a 2004 study in the *Journal of Studies on Alcohol,* in 2000 there were approximately 231 deaths in the United States as a result of alcohol poisoning, deaths that occurred because of binge drinking. Binge drinking and deaths from alcohol poisoning remain serious problems in the United States.

Fact or Fiction?

Drinking coffee is a good way to fight alcohol poisoning.

The Facts: It is true that the caffeine in coffee can help someone develop a slightly higher **tolerance** for alcohol. Research has shown that drinking coffee while drinking alcohol will allow a person to consume slightly more alcohol without becoming impaired. However, coffee has no ability to disrupt, prevent, or treat alcohol poisoning. When alcohol poisoning is a problem, the alcohol needs to be removed. Adding caffeine may help a person stay awake, but it will not treat the problem.

See also: Alcohol Abuse, The Risks of; Binge Drinking Among Teenagers; Effects of Alcohol on the Body

FURTHER READING
Cornett, Donna J. *7 Weeks to Safe Social Drinking.* Santa Rosa, Calif.: People Friendly Books, 2005.

■ BINGE DRINKING AMONG TEENAGERS

Not all people who study alcohol abuse use the term *binge drinking* the same way. However, the definition used by the National Household Survey on Drug Abuse (NHSDA) is a good place to start.

NHSDA defines binge drinking as consuming "five or more drinks on the same occasion on at least 1 day in the past 30 days. By 'occasion' is meant at the same time or within a couple of hours of each other." To the NHSDA, a "drink" is a 1.5-ounce shot of 80-proof liquor, a 12-ounce bottle of regular beer, or a five-ounce glass of wine.

WHAT IS BINGE DRINKING?

Alcohol can intoxicate some people after one or two drinks. Teenagers who have never had alcohol may experience that the first time they drink. Even many adults, if they only drink on special occasions, can get tipsy after just a couple of drinks.

Other people find it harder to get drunk and feel they have to work at it. You may ask: Does anybody really *try* to get drunk? According to data compiled in 2007 by Monitoring the Future, a project of the National Institute on Drug Abuse, most teenagers *don't*—only 28.7 percent had been drunk in the past 30 days. Also, although more than 40 percent of high school kids have been drunk at least once, they usually don't repeat the experience.

Unfortunately, however, some teenagers do make an effort to get drunk, and they do it time after time. Those people are binge drinkers—they have frequent episodes of drinking too much. This is the most widespread form of alcohol abuse among young Americans. According to the Youth Risk Behavior Surveillance System, some 26 percent of high school students in 2007 reported binge drinking in the previous month.

Some kids may binge once, suffer harmful or even disastrous consequences, and never do it again. Some other teens, usually older, can manage to have four or five drinks once in a while without causing serious harm to themselves or others and without becoming alcohol dependent. Some people would call them binge drinkers; others would not. But the experts agree that far too many teenagers in America have a serious problem with binge drinking. Thousands of kids are bingeing, and they are putting their lives and futures at risk.

The Harvard School of Public Health limits the term "binge drinker" to those who have had five or more drinks on one occasion in the past *two weeks* rather than 30 days. They use the five-drink cutoff point for men but lower it to four drinks for women, since women are more likely to become intoxicated, and suffer physical harm, with less alcohol. Using different standards makes it difficult to compare the results of different surveys.

The Higher Education Center for Alcohol and Other Drug Prevention, an agency of the U.S. Department of Education, deals with the very real problem of alcohol abuse on college campuses. In 2000, the center said that five drinks should not always be considered a binge. A better definition, it said, would take into account the drinker's body weight, as well as how fast he or she drinks and how much food he or she eats while drinking. All those factors change the impact of alcohol on the body and brain. College officials, the center said, found that students were dismissing messages against alcohol abuse, since they believed the definitions were unrealistic.

Fact Or Fiction?

*People who graduate from college drink more
than other Americans.*

The Facts: The above statement is a "half-truth." According to the National Survey on Drug Use and Health, 63.7 percent of college students ages 18 to 22 report drinking in the past month. An estimated 53.5 percent of people ages 18 to 22 who are not full-time college students report drinking in the past month. However, the research also shows that college graduates are less likely to engage in binge drinking or heavy alcohol use.

However they define the term, all these agencies find it useful to distinguish binge drinkers from heavy drinkers and **alcoholics**. "Bingers" do not necessarily progress to heavy drinking (usually defined as bingeing several times a month), and they may never feel the physical or emotional cravings that dominate the lives of alcoholics.

Teenage drinkers should not take too much comfort in this distinction. Anyone who deliberately drinks to the point of intoxication, even on just an occasional basis, is engaging in binge drinking, with all its risks. It is especially worrisome if he or she intends to do so again in the future.

Sometimes bingeing is obvious. Teenagers often tell therapists and counselors about "drinking games," in which one participant pours alcohol into another person's mouth directly from a bottle or through a funnel, in which teens take turns drinking directly from a beer keg, or in which kids swallow "Jell-O shots." These are obvious examples of binge drinking.

But binge drinking also occurs when a few young friends get into the habit of gathering every Sunday to watch an afternoon of ball games and drink one light beer after another until some or all of them are drunk. And of course, anyone who blacks out during drinking and cannot remember later some or all of what happened is bingeing dangerously.

HOW COMMON IS BINGEING?

Until experts agree on a definition, any numbers must be considered estimates. But the best estimates issued by government agencies offer

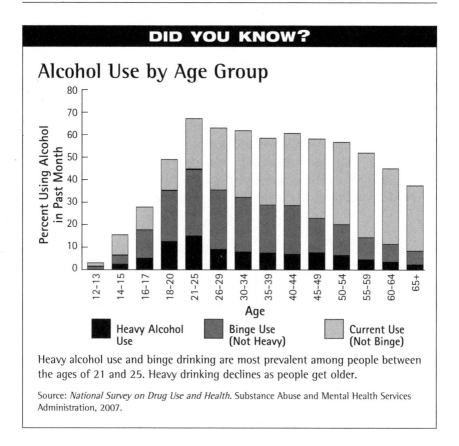

DID YOU KNOW?

Alcohol Use by Age Group

Heavy alcohol use and binge drinking are most prevalent among people between the ages of 21 and 25. Heavy drinking declines as people get older.

Source: *National Survey on Drug Use and Health.* Substance Abuse and Mental Health Services Administration, 2007.

both good and bad news. The good news is that teenage bingeing has declined in the last few years, and has declined even more as compared with 20 years ago. The bad news is, bingeing is still a major problem.

Monitoring the Future has some of the best data for binge drinking, which they also call heavy episodic drinking and which they define as five drinks or more in the past two weeks. They report that the practice had declined among 12th graders from 41 percent in 1983 to 28 percent in 1992. After rising for a while in the 1990s, it began declining again, and fell to 28.6 percent in 2002. By 2007, that dropped to 27 percent.

In addition, more 12th graders today seem to understand the risks involved in bingeing. In 1982, 36 percent believed that drinking heavily once or twice each weekend carried a "great risk"; the number rose to 49 percent in 1992. In 2007, 45.8 percent believed so.

In 2007, among eighth graders, 10.3 percent engaged in binge drinking. For 10th graders, 21.9 percent engaged in binge drinking, while 25.9 percent of 12th graders admitted to binge drinking.

Monitoring the Future reported figures for binge drinking among various subgroups within the grades. In 2007, for eighth graders, the gender breakdown was 10.4 percent for boys and 10.0 for girls. The racial breakdown was 15.6 percent for Hispanic Americans, 7.7 percent for African Americans, and 9.7 percent for Caucasians.

The greatest contrasts involved the parents' education level. Nearly 19 percent of the eighth graders whose parents did not complete high school binged, while only 6.2 percent of those whose parents attended graduate school did so. For 10th and 12th graders, the gender and racial breakdowns were similar, but the effect of parents' education and kids' college plans became much less important.

For Americans as a whole, binge drinking seems to peak at age 21 and declines as the age group advances. This suggests that the majority of people who binge as kids "outgrow" the experience. Unfortunately, some get stuck along the way, with serious consequences.

RISKS

The American Psychological Association reported in 2001 that according to the latest evidence, heavy drinking by teens might do more damage to their nervous systems than had been thought. According to these studies, the human brain continues to develop until the age of 21. As a result, "teens who binge drink may do damage to their memory and learning abilities by severely hampering the development of the hippocampus." (This small but important part of the brain has a major role in storing memories and regulating motivation.)

Of course, most of the behavioral risks that pertain to alcohol abuse apply to binge drinking. Bingers are responsible for a large proportion of DWI motor vehicle accidents involving teens. The more frequent and intense the binges, the more drinkers are likely to also engage in risky sex, injure themselves, and be victims of violent crimes. The outward physical effects of bingeing, such as extreme intoxication or passing out in public, also ensure that teenage bingers have a good chance of getting in trouble with the law.

Binge drinking can also sometimes lead to alcohol **dependency**. It is not true, as some people mistakenly believe, that you can't become an alcoholic if you drink only on weekends. Several studies have found that high school binge drinkers are very likely to binge drink in college as well, according to a 1995 report from the National Institute of Alcohol Abuse and Alcoholism. This type of behavior pattern, which lasts for several years, can become hard to break, even though high school and college bingers often do not believe they are problem drinkers.

SECONDHAND EFFECTS OF BINGEING

Teenagers are notorious for thinking they are "immortal." Even when they fully understand the dangers of risky behavior, they sometimes find it hard to believe that "it could happen to me." If you are one of those teens, then at least consider the real risk that if you binge, you may harm other people. Innocent bystanders who do not voluntarily assume the risk often become the victims.

Motor vehicle accidents do the most damage, but binge drinking affects other secondhand victims too. The authors of a 2008 article in the *Journal of Studies on Alcohol and Drugs* discuss the secondhand effect of binge drinking. According to the authors, in areas where there is a high rate of binge drinking, the local residents are more likely to experience problems with noise, property damage, and police visits.

LEARN THE FACTS

Despite attempts to educate kids to the dangers of binge drinking, teenage bingeing remains a serious problem in the United States. Kids need to learn the facts in order to be able to make the intelligent choice when the situation arises.

See also: Alcohol Abuse, The Risks of; Drinking on College Campuses

FURTHER READING

Hyde, Margaret O., and John F. Setaro. *Alcohol 101: An Overview for Teens.* Bookfield, Conn.: Twenty-first Century, 1999.

Stewart, Gail B. *Teen Alcoholics.* San Diego, Calif.: Lucent, 2000.

Torr, James D. ed. *Alcoholism.* San Diego, Calif.: Greenhaven, 2000.

Volkmann, Chris, and Toren Volkmann. *From Binge to Blackout: A Mother and Son Struggle with Teen Drinking.* New York: New American Library, 2006.

■ BIRTH DEFECTS AND ALCOHOL

A birth defect is a health problem that develops while the baby is forming inside the mother. The defect may be inherited or acquired. One of the leading causes of birth defects, mental retardation, and developmental disabilities in children is also 100 percent preventable—drinking during pregnancy. Yet every year, one in 30 pregnant women indulges in risk drinking that may damage her baby.

Risk drinking is defined as seven or more drinks per week (also called frequent drinking or heavy drinking), or five or more drinks on one occasion (called binge drinking). Another one in seven women of childbearing age, who is pregnant but not aware of it, also engages in risk drinking.

The range of alcohol-related birth defects and disabilities runs the spectrum from mild learning and social problems to profound retardation. The most severe form of alcohol-related disorder is **fetal alcohol syndrome,** commonly known as FAS.

FETAL ALCOHOL SYNDROME

When a pregnant mother drinks, the alcohol in her bloodstream easily crosses the placenta, an organ in most mammals that connects the developing fetus to the mother's uterus and enters her baby's system through the umbilical cord. While scientists are still not sure exactly how alcohol damages a baby in utero (that is, in the mother's uterus or womb), they do know that FAS, the severest form of alcohol-related birth defects, is most frequently associated with frequent or heavy drinking, binge drinking, and alcoholism.

FAS is actually a group of alcohol-related birth abnormalities that primarily affect three areas: the face, the brain, and growth.

Facial abnormalities

Many children with FAS have a distinctive facial appearance, which may include any of the following: a small head; widely spaced eyes with epicanthic folds (an elongation of the fold in the upper eyelids); a low nasal bridge and flat midface; a short nose; minor ear abnormalities; a thin upper lip; or a narrowed jaw. These facial abnormalities occur during the first trimester (first three months) of pregnancy.

Facial, organ, and bone damage generally happen because of drinking during the first trimester of pregnancy. During the third and fourth week of this trimester, the embryo's arms, central nervous system, eyes, heart, and legs are developing and are especially vulnerable to damage.

Brain abnormalities

FAS-related brain and central nervous system abnormalities can occur throughout pregnancy and may include moderate to severe mental retardation; low IQ; developmental delays; speech and language delays; behavior disorders; and poor learning, memory, and problem-solving skills.

The brain of the unborn child develops throughout pregnancy, during all three trimesters, so brain damage related to alcohol can happen at any time during pregnancy.

Growth abnormalities

Infants born with FAS are often significantly underweight and smaller than other newborns, putting them at greater risk for lung and heart failure, and for viral and bacterial infections during the newborn period. They also may have skeletal abnormalities, organ defects, and hearing problems. As children, they are generally smaller in stature and slower to grow than unaffected children and may have poor coordination and muscle control. These FAS-related growth effects can occur throughout pregnancy. However, alcohol-related low birth weight and smaller-than-average size are most associated with drinking during the *third* trimester (last three months) of pregnancy.

Q & A

Question: My friend told me it's okay to drink when I'm pregnant. What amount of alcohol is safe to drink?

Answer: *No* amount of alcohol is safe to drink during pregnancy—or if you are trying to *get* pregnant, since many women do not know that they are pregnant for three to eight weeks after conception. While frequent or heavy drinking, alcoholic drinking, and binge drinking are most associated with severe damage to the unborn child, any alcohol consumed increases the chances of a child being born with physical, learning, and behavioral problems. Despite what some people believe, there is no "safe time" to drink during pregnancy.

Prevalence of FAS

Scientists do not know the exact prevalence of FAS. (*Prevalence* refers to the percentage of a population affected by a disease or disorder at a given time.) Prevalence rates found vary by type of research study done and by populations studied. Studies by the Centers for Disease Control and Prevention (CDC) in the 1990s have found FAS prevalence rates between 0.2 and 1.5 per 1,000 live births in different areas of the country. Rates as high as three per 1,000 live births have been found among some populations. These figures roughly translate to several thousand babies born in the United States with FAS each year.

Fact Or Fiction?

Any drinking during pregnancy causes birth defects.

The Facts: Many women and their babies are vulnerable to alcohol's toxic effects, even when they drink only small quantities, but the truth is, some women can drink during a pregnancy and have healthy babies. And this is good news for the many healthy babies born to mothers who drink during pregnancy. But it is bad news for maternal and child health care advocates who work hard to educate young women about the dangers of drinking during pregnancy. Scientists do not know why this is true, and they cannot predict which women and babies are most susceptible. The bottom line is: The only sure way to protect your baby from alcohol-related birth defects is not to drink.

OTHER ALCOHOL-RELATED BIRTH DISORDERS

Although full-blown FAS is a profoundly damaging disorder, it is relatively rare. However, other very serious alcohol-related birth disorders occur with greater frequency.

Many children diagnosed with FAS have a distinctly less severe form of the condition. Other children exposed to their mothers' drinking during pregnancy have some (but not all) of the symptoms of FAS. In the past, scientists used the general term "fetal alcohol effects" (FAE) to describe the FAS-like disorders of both groups of children. Currently, most researchers use two other terms, which more clearly define FAE: alcohol-related neurodevelopmental disorder (ARND) and alcohol-related birth defects (ARBD).

ARND refers to the mental, learning, and behavioral problems experienced by a child exposed to a mother's alcohol use during pregnancy. Symptoms include poor academic performance; impaired mathematical skills; alcohol-related attention deficit hyperactivity disorder (ADHD); other attention, judgment, and impulse disorders; memory impairment; and poor emotional control.

ARBD is used to describe alcohol-caused physical defects and includes deformities of the face, skull, skeleton, and auditory system, as well as defects in the heart, kidneys, and other organs.

The prevalence of ARND and ARBD (together often called FAE) is far greater than FAS but more difficult to estimate because the disorders are frequently harder to diagnose as alcohol-related.

THE COSTS OF FAS AND FAE

FAS and FAE are incurable disorders that affect a child physically, intellectually, emotionally, and behaviorally throughout his or her life. The impact on the child's family, which invariably needs much outside support, is also huge and lasts a lifetime. These kinds of costs are immeasurable.

The economic costs associated with FAS and FAE are estimated at nearly $3 billion a year. The average lifetime cost of treating one person with FAS or FAE is $3 million and includes monies spent for counseling; the criminal justice, prison, and welfare systems; family outreach programs; health care; and special education.

HELP SPREAD THE WORD

Fortunately, the message has gotten out to most people: Drinking during pregnancy can have devastating consequences for the woman and for her child. Birth defects are always heart breaking; when they could have been prevented, they are tragic. Teens can and should do their part to spread the word and help eliminate FAS from their society.

See also: Alcohol and Disease; Alcoholism, Causes of; Binge Drinking Among Teenagers; Sexual Behavior and Alcohol

FURTHER READING

Kulp, Liz. *The Best I Can Be: Living with Fetal Alcohol Syndrome Effects.* Brooklyn Park, Minn.: Better Endings New Beginnings, 2000.

Nevitt, Amy. *Fetal Alcohol Syndrome.* New York: Rosen Publishing Group, 1996.

Soby, Jeanette M. *Prenatal Exposure to Drugs/Alcohol: Characteristics and Educational Implications of Fetal Alcohol Syndrome and Cocaine/polydrug Effects.* Springfield, Ill.: Charles C. Thomas Publisher, 2006.

■ CAUSES OF ALCOHOLISM
See: Alcoholism, Causes of

■ CHILDREN AND ALCOHOL
See: Birth Defects and Alcohol; Underage Drinking

■ CHILDREN OF ALCOHOLICS
If you turned to this section first, you may be wondering if one of your parents (or another adult relative or caretaker) is an **alcoholic.** Here's a simple test; answer yes or no to the following statements:

- ■ I often wish my dad or mom would cut down on or stop his or her drinking.
- ■ I often feel angry about my dad's or mom's drinking.
- ■ I often feel guilty about my dad's or mom's drinking, as if I were to blame.
- ■ I am afraid or embarrassed to bring friends home because my dad or mom might be drunk.

If you answered yes to one of these questions, chances are that your mom, dad, or other adult caretaker has a drinking problem and may be an alcoholic. You are not alone. Nearly 11 million children and teenagers in the United States are growing up in alcoholic families, according to SAMHSA, the federal Substance Abuse and Mental Health Services Administration.

Alcoholism experts who study children of alcoholics—COAs for short—believe that they are at a higher risk than children of nonalcoholics (non-COAs) for having a variety of emotional and learning problems and for becoming alcoholics themselves.

COAS AND THE RISK OF EMOTIONAL PROBLEMS

COAs are at greater risk than non-COAs to suffer from depression, anxiety disorders, and psychiatric or developmental problems that require medication or hospitalization, such as attention deficit hyperactivity disorder (ADHD), a syndrome in some children characterized by inattention, impulsiveness, and hyperactivity, and oppositional defiant disorder (ODD), a related syndrome of socially disruptive behavioral problems.

COAs may also experience more intense feelings of anger, confusion, embarrassment, guilt, and isolation than do non-COAs. They may be more aggressive than other children, complain frequently about headaches and stomachaches, skip school, and engage in risk-taking behaviors.

COAS AND THE RISK OF LEARNING PROBLEMS

According to a 1997 report in *Alcohol Health and Research World,* some research studies believe that COAs and non-COAs differ most in the area of thinking and learning, called cognitive function by experts. Their research suggests that while most COAs fall within normal ranges on intelligence (IQ) tests, they may have lower scores on IQ arithmetic, reading, and verbal tests than non-COAs.

COAs also have lower scores on performance tests that measure abstract and conceptual thinking. The authors of a 2008 article in *Family Relations* found that adult children of alcoholics have poorer behavioral control than those who did not have alcoholic parents. In particular, the authors focused on the ability of adult COAs to use higher-order thinking to help regulate behavior. In a similar vein, the authors of a 2008 article in *Social Psychiatry and Psychiatric Epidemiology* also found that ACOAs had lower cognitive functioning.

COAS AND THE RISK OF ALCOHOLISM— GENETICS OR ENVIRONMENT?

COAs are considered the highest-risk group for becoming alcoholics (and drug abusers), and genetics (a person's inherited characteristics or features) is a big factor. Biological children of alcoholics who are adopted by nonalcoholics still have a two- to nine-fold greater risk of becoming alcoholics, despite not being raised in an alcoholic environment.

Compared to non-COAs, COAs have four times the risk of becoming alcoholics, according to SAMHSA. Sons of alcoholic fathers have an even greater risk for alcohol abuse, and they become alcoholics at an earlier age than their sisters.

Genetics, however, is only part of the problem. Environment also helps determine whether or not COAs go on to abuse alcohol themselves. The alcoholic family environment is a chaotic and uncertain one at best. Poor parenting, marital and financial problems, poor relations between siblings, and the disruption of significant events, such as birthdays and holidays, can all combine to put enormous stress on COAs. Add to that the pressure of adolescence, school, friends, dating, and society in general. Is it any wonder that many children of alcoholics, with a lack of caring support, are especially vulnerable to drinking and alcohol abuse?

THE "ROLES" COAS PLAY IN THEIR FAMILIES

Early research about COAs focused on the unique personalities adopted as coping mechanisms by children living with alcoholism—especially those with siblings (brothers and sisters). Researchers identified four main roles that most COAs play in their families in response to the chaos and uncertainty alcoholism breeds. However, many of today's researchers believe these early COA labels are too broad and do not take into account the fact that every alcoholic family—and every COA—is unique.

Still, many self-help books continue to use these terms, which can be useful for looking at your own response to an alcoholic parent. Do you recognize any of these classic COA roles?

- The **hero or heroine,** usually the oldest child, who takes over many of the caretaking responsibilities of the alcoholic parent and who excels in school and sports;

- The **scapegoat,** often the second oldest child, who assumes the role of angry troublemaker to get the attention he or she feel deserving of and who is most likely to use alcohol and drugs at an early age;

- The **lost or quiet child,** usually a middle child, who tries never to cause any trouble, is often sad and withdrawn and has a tendency to be sickly; and

■ The **mascot or clown,** frequently the youngest child in the family, who uses humor and clowning around to focus attention on himself or herself to try to diffuse the tension and anger in the family and who is most likely to need psychiatric help later in life.

Many COAs are not destined to be troubled teens or alcoholics. In fact, more than half of COAs studied by researchers lead normal, healthy, successful lives and never become alcohol dependent. The experts call this group resilient COAs, and they share many common characteristics.

THE RESILIENT COA

More than anything else, resilient COAs believe in self-help and know how to ask for help. They reach out to caring adults outside the family—for example, a relative, a friend's parent, a teacher, or a coach—with whom they can share their feelings and get support and advice. Resilient COAs are also good communicators, have a caring attitude toward others, and have a real desire to achieve. They make it a priority to get and stay active in school, sports, and the community. They seek out support groups where they can talk to other teens who share similar problems and ambitions.

Are you a resilient COA? If so, remember the first rule of survival: Resilient people know they cannot "do it" alone—they ask for help.

Q & A

Question: My father's been an alcoholic all my life. Does that mean I'll be an alcoholic too?

Answer: No, it doesn't, but you are right to be concerned. Children of alcoholics (COAs) are four times more likely than non-COAs to become addicted to alcohol if they decide to drink, and the sons of alcoholic fathers are at particular risk. Your best defense is to learn about alcoholism and the signs of addiction, look for help and support outside the family, and—most importantly—not drink!

IT'S NOT YOUR FAULT!

Many COAs believe that they are the cause of their parent's drinking, or that they can control or cure a parent's alcoholism if they behave a certain way—by getting better grades, for example, or by being a superstar on the soccer field or helping out more around the house. Sadly, many alcoholics often encourage this kind of thinking through their tendency to blame others, including their children, for their drinking problems. But children must remember that they are NOT to blame, and *no one* can "cure" alcoholism. Your parent has to want to stop drinking and has to ask for help. In the meantime, you have to take care of yourself.

The National Association for Children of Alcoholics (NACOA) suggests you start taking care of yourself by remembering the "Seven Cs":

- I didn't   CAUSE it.
- I can't   CURE it.
- I can't   CONTROL it.
- I can take better CARE of myself
- by   COMMUNICATING my feelings,
- making healthy   CHOICES,
- and   CELEBRATING myself.

GETTING HELP

Information equals power! The following books and Web sites provide a range of information about alcoholism and growing up in an alcoholic family and offer suggestions for where to go to get help.

THE GOOD NEWS

Many children of alcoholics start life with a definite handicap. They may be justified in feeling angry or resentful at times. Fortunately, the clear majority of COAs overcome their disadvantages—and their resentments—and manage to build decent lives for themselves. They have broken the cycle, thereby freeing their own future children from the burden of an alcoholic family.

See also: Alcoholism, Causes of; Depression and Alcohol; Recovery and Treatment; Self-Help Programs

FURTHER READING

Alateen—Hope for Children of Alcoholics. New York: Al-Anon Family Group Headquarters, Inc., 1980.

Carrick, Carol. *Banana Bear.* Morton Grove, Ill.: Albert Whitman and Company, 1995.

Hornik-Beer, Edith Lynn. *For Teenagers with a Parent Who Abuses Alcohol/Drugs.* Lincoln, Neb.: iUniverse.com, Inc., 2001.

Petit, Roland. *Transformation for Life: Healing and Growth for Adult Children of Alcoholics and Others.* Watertown, Mass.: Bright Horizons Press, 2005.

Langsen, Richard, and Nicole Rubel. *When Someone in the Family Drinks Too Much.* New York: Dial Books for Young Readers, 1996.

■ CHOICES, RESPONSIBLE

Decisions mindful of both positive and negative consequences. Some teens will decide not to drink at all. After all, millions of Americans manage to live normal lives with little or no alcohol. They abstain for reasons of health, religion, morality, or just personal preference.

However, teens who plan to drink can learn how to bypass the dangerous phase of alcohol abuse that other teens and young adults go through. If careful, they can learn how to drink safely *without* having to "learn from their mistakes"—some of which can be costly.

Alcohol has been a part of life since before the dawn of civilization. When abused, it has been a source of hostility and aggression, disease and early death, poverty and divorce, accidents and economic loss. But it has also helped millions overcome shyness and social inhibition; strengthen bonds with friends, relatives, and colleagues; or just relax and have a good time.

The majority of American adults, adding up the pluses and the minuses, have decided to drink. According to the 2007 National Household Survey on Drug Abuse, more than 68.3 percent of Americans between the ages of 21 and 25 had a drink in the previous month. Older age groups were a little less likely to imbibe, but not by much—47.6 percent of Americans aged 60–64 had a drink in the previous month, according to the same survey.

But buried in the mountain of statistics that the Household Survey gathers, one interesting fact stands out: While many young adults drink heavily, as people mature their heavy drinking and binge drinking decline.

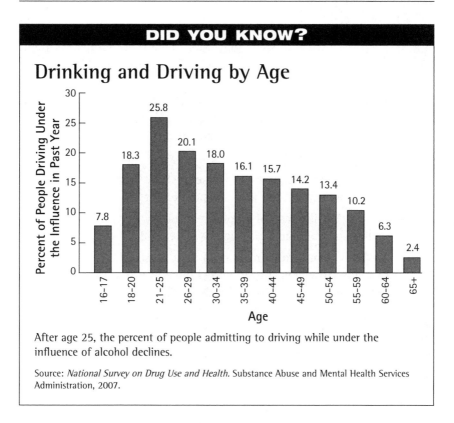

Drinking and Driving by Age

After age 25, the percent of people admitting to driving while under the influence of alcohol declines.

Source: *National Survey on Drug Use and Health.* Substance Abuse and Mental Health Services Administration, 2007.

Although only a small proportion of children 12–17 years old drank heavily, the numbers changed dramatically for the 18–25 age group, more than a third of whom were binge drinkers. Yet every age group older than 25 had smaller and smaller numbers of heavy and binge drinkers, even though the total number of alcohol users remained largely the same. By the time they were in their thirties, the solid majority of Americans who used alcohol had become moderate drinkers. They had learned to enjoy a limited amount of alcohol, without drinking enough to cause harm.

RESPONSIBLE DRINKING

A simple phrase has become popular in recent decades: "responsible drinking." It encompasses all the commonsense rules, detailed in this entry, that keep drinkers from harming themselves or others.

There are two ways of approaching responsible drinking—as a goal, and as a means to get to that goal. Most people agree on the goal, but they may differ about how to reach it—especially on how to help teenagers reach it.

Nearly 30 years ago, the National Institute for Alcohol Abuse and Alcoholism (NIAAA), in a report to the U.S. Congress, came up with a series of guidelines designed to encourage responsible drinking behavior. It read as follows:

- Alcohol is a drug that can cause positive and negative social, psychological, and physical effects.
- The responsible use of alcohol can be socially, psychologically, and physically beneficial.
- To drink or not to drink should be a personal decision. However, those who choose to drink have a responsibility not to damage themselves or society.
- People who drink need to respect the decision of those who do not drink.
- People who serve alcoholic beverages need to contribute to a healthy drinking environment and not "push" drinks on others.
- Intoxication is not responsible drinking. There is a direct link between responsible attitudes toward drinking and the alleviation of the problem of alcohol.

Almost everyone agrees with these principles. A lot of lives could be saved if Americans learned to take them to heart—and put them into practice. Yet principles need to be fleshed out with details: What should people learn to do, and not to do?

The oldest approach to alcohol education is to accentuate the negative. Most states have required alcohol education in the public schools for many years, often going back to the days of the **temperance movement,** when many Americans believed all drinking was immoral. For 14 years early in the 20th century (1919–33), all drinking was illegal too.

As a result, the traditional education curriculum has focused on the harm alcohol can do to the body and on the devastating effects of alcoholism on individuals and their families. Of course, teenagers do need to understand these facts. But they do not live in a vacuum.

They know that most of their parents drink, and they can guess that many of their teachers drink too. They see alcohol served in most of the restaurants they patronize. Even if their parents abstain, they know through TV and movies that drinking is commonplace in America.

As a result, many educators now believe that the negative approach may not be the most effective with teenagers. Kids tend to shy away from lessons that sound like preaching—"Do as I say, not as I do" is a good way to turn off kids. Instead, some educators suggest, these teenagers should be clearly taught that drinking in moderation is an acceptable choice for adults, just as **abstinence** (not drinking at all) is an acceptable choice. They also should be taught what "drinking in moderation" really means.

David Hanson, a psychologist and alcohol educator at the State University of New York, is a strong advocate of teaching young people the rules of sensible drinking. He writes, "Teaching about responsible use does not require student consumption of alcohol, any more than teaching them world geography requires them to visit Nepal."

In that spirit, the following section describes the main rules of responsible alcohol use.

Know what you are drinking

Learn about the different alcohol contents of popular beverages. Wine sold in the United States has the percent alcohol listed on the label. Liquor labels show the "proof"; divide by two to get the percent. But be careful: Liquor bought outside the United States may list the percent; multiply the percent by two to get the proof. As a rule of thumb, a can or bottle of beer has the same amount of alcohol as a glass of wine or a shot of liquor. Act accordingly: If two shots of whiskey get you drunk, so do two beers.

You may not see the label if you are served by a waiter or a host. Be aware that a 12-ounce serving of ale typically has one-third more alcohol than the same amount of light beer; sherry has 50 percent more alcohol than the same amount of red wine; and bourbon may have 50 percent more alcohol by weight than most scotch whiskies.

If you are offered a premixed drink, find out what's inside. A cup of fruit punch may taste like a soft drink but may contain the alcohol equivalent of one or more shots of liquor. If you don't trust the judgment of the person who is pouring, pour your own drink—or drink something less "suspicious."

Pace yourself
Remember, your body can only process one standard-size drink in an hour. Sip your drink slowly. Dilute liquor with noncarbonated mixers, water, or ice. When your drink is getting low, add some more mixer or ice. If you feel drunk, stop drinking; or better yet, order a nonalcoholic beverage to help dilute the alcohol in your system. Always keep track of the number of drinks you've had—you can easily forget, when you are intoxicated.

Know your capacity
Women do not process alcohol as quickly as men. They can drink a lot less and still be "keeping up." The same is true for men or women who weigh less than average.

Choose the right time and place
Do not drink by yourself or when you are feeling tired, unwell, or unhappy. Try to drink only with people you like, in a pleasant atmosphere. Never drink on an empty stomach.

Don't drink for the wrong reasons
Don't ever drink to be polite, to be one of the crowd, or to show off.

Don't drink and drive
Don't drink and drive or drink and operate heavy machinery.

ABSTINENCE
Millions of Americans are quiet abstainers. You would not know from the mass media, but a huge proportion of adult Americans never drinks alcohol at all. The 2006 National Health Interview Survey revealed that 25 percent of people of drinking age in the United States have never had a drink.

For all practical purposes, people who almost never drink can be considered "abstainers." In fact, that's what the NIAAA calls anyone who never has more than 12 drinks in a single year.

People abstain for a variety of reasons. About two million recovering alcoholics choose not to have even one drink, for fear of risking a relapse into addiction. Some of their children also abstain, having seen firsthand the negative aspects of alcohol. Many other Americans have health conditions or take medications that make drinking alcohol dangerous or harmful. Others do not like the taste of alcohol, or enjoy the feeling of being even mildly "high."

Many more abstain out of principle. Some organic or health food fans consider any drugs, including caffeine and alcohol, to be contrary to their ideas of fitness and nutrition. Also, many athletes believe alcohol impairs their performance.

Some religious denominations either ban alcohol outright or frown on its use. These groups include some long-established American churches such as the Baptists, Mormons, and Pentecostalists, as well as communities of Muslims, Buddhists, and Hindus. The reasons they give for abstinence vary, but they share the goal of avoiding harm to their followers and society.

MAKE THE RIGHT CHOICE FOR YOU

The abuse of alcohol embitters the lives of millions of Americans. Yet even more millions have learned how to deal with this powerful substance by abstaining or drinking responsibly. You can learn too; a few intelligent choices today can save you years of trouble in the future.

See also: Binge Drinking Among Teenagers; Law and Drinking, The

FURTHER READING
Claypool, Jane. *Alcohol and You.* New York: Grolier, 1997.
Cornett, D.J. *Seven Weeks to Safe Social Drinking: How to Effectively Moderate Your Alcohol Intake.* Secaucus, N.J.: Carol Publishing Group, 1997.
Rotgers, Frederick, Marc F. Kern, and Rudy Hoeltzel. *Responsible Drinking: A Moderation Management Approach for Problem Drinkers.* Oakland, Calif.: New Harbinger Publications, 2002.

■ CODEPENDENCY

An unhealthy and usually unspoken relationship between an alcoholic and nonalcoholic significant other or family member who unwittingly supports the alcoholic's behavior. Sometimes the supporting member even pretends the **addiction** to alcohol does not exist.

A codependent relationship is **dysfunctional**. It consists of a problem drinker and a partner. The codependency is found in the partner. Because of low self-esteem, or other psychological issues, the partner stays in the relationship and often helps enable the problem drinking.

Although codependency was once an important topic of discussion, some scholars now question the usefulness of the concept; they point out there are few validated tools to screen for codependency. Instead, they argue that the focus should be on **enabling behaviors** and how partners cope with the stressful situation.

CHARACTERISTICS OF CODEPENDENCY

Certain groups of people are believed to be at a high risk for developing a codependent relationship. These are people who are involved with someone with a **substance abuse** disorder. Although the term *codependency* once focused on the problematic relationship between an alcoholic and his or her partner, today it refers to all relationships in which someone has a substance abuse issue—with alcohol, illegal drugs, prescription drugs, or any other chemical.

A key feature of a codependent is the need to be needed. Such people do not have enough self-esteem to feel worthwhile as they are. Their self-esteem is dependent on how others view them. According to the National Council on Alcoholism and Drug Abuse in St. Louis, there are several problems exhibited by those with a codependence experience. These include

- difficulty in accurately identifying and expressing feelings
- rigidity in behavior and/or attitudes
- feeling overly responsible for other people's behavior and feelings
- feeling powerless
- a basic sense of shame and low self-esteem
- difficulty in forming or maintaining close relationships

One aspect of codependency is enabling behavior. Some experts believe that enabling is the better concept on which to focus. To enable a person is to help that person do something. In this case, however, the "help" is negative reinforcement; enabling refers to behaviors that help someone continue with an addiction. This includes facilitating behavior and avoiding the negative consequences of the behavior.

The authors of a 2008 study in the *American Journal of Orthopsychiatry* examined codependence in women in Mexico City seeking primary-care treatment with their doctors. The authors found that women who had partners with suspected alcohol dependence were 4.7 times more likely to display signs of codependence than women without such partners. The authors also found that women were 1.9 times more likely to develop signs of codependence if their fathers had had drinking problems. Also, women with abusive partners were 3.6 times more likely to shows signs of codependence compared to women without abusive partners.

Q & A

Question: Do most relationships where alcohol and substance abuse are a problem involve some form of aggression?

Answer: Yes, relationships where substance abuse, including alcohol, is a problem are more likely to involve both psychological and physical aggression. For example, the authors of a 2008 study in *Drug and Alcohol Dependence* examined instances of aggression in relationships where substance abuse existed. They found that the substance abuser engaged in psychological aggression in 77 percent of relationships, while physical aggression occurred in 54 percent of the relationships. The partners were also aggressive: 73 percent of them engaged in psychological aggression against the substance abuser, and 51 percent of them engaged in physical aggression.

The authors of a 2000 study in the *Archives of Psychiatric Nursing* examined codependency among elderly women. This is one of the few studies that has focused exclusively on women ages 65 and older. It was discovered, once again, that there is a relationship between codependency and depression. Further, there was a negative relationship between codependency and both perceived health and ability to function. In other words, women believed they were less healthy and less likely to function properly on a daily basis if they displayed stronger indications of codependency.

PREDICTORS OF CODEPENDENCY

Results of a 1999 study in the *Journal of Clinical Psychology* indicate that low self-confidence is an excellent predictor of codependence. The authors also suggested that future studies should further explore the differences between low self-confidence and codependence.

There is also some research that shows a relationship between codependency and having a codependent parent. According to a study in the *Journal of Clinical Psychology,* however, it is hard to determine exactly why a codependent relationship exists. Although codependency could be a learned behavior, the authors also suggested that exposure to codependency, combined with unhealthy parenting styles, puts a child at risk for becoming codependent in adulthood.

ENABLING BEHAVIORS

A 2004 study in the *Journal of Substance Abuse Treatment* focused on specific behaviors that enabled a significant other to continue with problematic drinking. The authors found that 41 out of the 42 people in the study engaged in some form of enabling behavior. The most common forms of enabling were lying to friends and family to cover up the problem and performing the partner's chores. In both cases, 69 percent of partners engaged in these behaviors. Sixty-seven percent threatened to leave their partner, but they never did. However, only 30 percent of people gave their partners money to buy alcohol. Finally, people were asked about their beliefs about their partner and his or her behaviors. The belief that "my partner can't get along without my help" was a significant predictor of engaging in enabling behavior.

Some research indicates that enabling behavior may be a coping mechanism as opposed to an element of codependency. For example, the authors of a 2008 study in *Family Relations* argue that women have been socialized to take care of their family. Instead of being codependent on the alcoholic partner, the woman views it as her job to take care of the partner. Interviews with women supported this interpretation. Each viewed her situation as a result of circumstances rather than her personality being drawn to a needy partner. Further, the women wanted to strive for normalcy in an abnormal situation. This can be interpreted as a normal reaction to a stressful situation, or a type of coping mechanism.

A 2006 study published in *Alcoholism Treatment Quarterly* also supports this interpretation of enabling behavior as a coping aid. The author interviewed people over the age of 10 in 18 families where a member was seeking counseling for problem drinking. Results indicated that family members, including an alcoholic's partner, worried about confronting the problem out of fear of alienating the person. They wanted to make the situation better, not worse. Many respondents were afraid they would lose their tempers, making a volatile situation even worse.

RECOVERING FROM CODEPENDENCY

Those who are codependent can recover from this problem. According to the Florida Alcohol and Drug Abuse Association (FADAA), there are four stages to recovering from codependency. They are

1. Denial
2. Acceptance
3. Core issues
4. Reintegration

The denial stage is straightforward—the person does not admit there is a problem. There may even be recognition that he or she should leave the relationship. However, the denial is so strong that it overrides the logical notion to leave.

Q & A

Question: Can couples get counseling to strengthen the relationship and eliminate codependency issues?

Answer: Couples counseling can indeed mitigate a codependent relationship. One approach that has had good success is Behavioral Couples Therapy (BCT). The goals of BCT are to help the person with the substance-abuse problem develop new coping skills to abstain from drugs and alcohol and to help partners cope with drinking-related situations. These two goals will help the relationship improve.

The results of a 2008 study in *Clinical Psychology Review* indicate that BCT helps improve the codependent relationship. However, the approach was not significantly more effective than individual counseling when it came to reducing substance use. This means that individual counseling is just as effective for treating the individual problems, while BCT helps address the relationship issues.

The acceptance stage in recovering from codependency is equally straightforward: The person acknowledges there is a problem and a need to fix it. It is at this stage when a person takes responsibility for the problem and the desire to change it. The core issues stage is common in psychological counseling for all types of issues. In this stage, the person accepts that it is impossible to control the actions and thoughts of others. Even though more than one person is involved in a codependent relationship, the person can only change his or her own behavior. It is up to the others in the relationship to change their behavior. In the reintegration stage, the last stage, people accept they are worthwhile and do not need to prove their worthiness to others.

PROBLEMS WITH CODEPENDENCY

Codependency, some have argued, has a negative connotation. In a way, it is considered a form of victim-blaming. This has been especially troublesome to feminist scholars because most victims of codependency are women.

Another problem is measuring codependency. Simply "knowing it when you see it" does not suffice when experts try to provide social and psychological help. Just as there are assessments to determine if someone has a drinking problem, there must be assessments to determine whether codependency exists and the extent of the problem. The few tools available have not been researched thoroughly enough to comfortably claim that they are completely reliable in identifying a codependent relationship. Without proper measures of codependency, it is difficult to say whether a person needs to be treated for the condition. Instead, it is better to avoid enabling behaviors and to help family members who may be problem drinkers face the consequences of their actions.

See also: Children of Alcoholics; Recovery and Treatment; Self-Help Programs

FURTHER READING

Beattie, Melody. *The New Codependency.* New York: Simon & Schuster, 2008.

Bryant-Jefferies, Richard. *Counseling the Person Beyond the Alcohol Problem.* Philadelphia: Jeesica Kingsley Publishers, 2009.

■ DISEASES ASSOCIATED WITH ALCOHOL
See: Alcohol and Disease

■ DRINKING AND DRIVING

Being a new driver isn't easy. Driving comes with hundreds of rules and regulations. Experience is the best teacher, which takes a lot of time and practice.

Saying no to the social pressure to drink isn't always easy either. Some of your friends are beginning to drink—some of them may have been experimenting with alcohol since grade school or even middle school. They may have a couple of beers or wine coolers before a dance, during a party, or after a football game. They look and act as if they are having a great time and may not seem drunk. And they want you to join in.

Do you? Can you say no? If saying no were an easy choice, few teenagers would struggle with it. Yet they do. By the time 12-year-olds have reached the sixth grade, almost 50 percent of them have been pressured into having a drink. So what do you do, especially if you are driving? Stop a minute, think, and consider these powerful facts.

DRIVING UNDER THE INFLUENCE (DUI)

Drinking and driving, or driving under the influence (DUI), means that the driver operates a motor vehicle while *under the influence* of alcohol. Sometimes this condition is referred to as driving while intoxicated (DWI).

Every state sets a maximum **BAC,** or **blood alcohol concentration,** limit for drivers over which it is considered unsafe—and against the law—to drive. If you are stopped for suspected drinking and driving, your BAC will be assessed. If you exceed your state's legal limit, you can be arrested and charged with driving under the influence or driving while intoxicated.

The authorities take DUI and DWI very seriously. You (or your parents, if you are under 21) will have to pay a fine. Your driver's license will be suspended for a set amount of time or, in some cases, completely revoked. If you are under 21, you also may not be allowed to get a new driver's license until you reach that age. And you may have to do community service as well as attend a special driver's education program. Also, the cost of your insurance will increase greatly.

DID YOU KNOW?

Drivers and Motorcycle Riders Involved in Fatal Crashes, by Age and Driver's Blood Alcohol Concentration (BAC)

Driver's BAC

Age (Years)	.00	.01–.07	.08 or higher	.01 or higher	
	Percent	Percent	Percent	Percent	Percent
<16	83	6	12	17	100
16–20	77	5	18	23	100
21–24	59	6	35	41	100
25–34	66	5	29	34	100
35–44	72	4	25	28	100
45–54	76	4	20	24	100
55–64	85	3	12	15	100
65–74	90	3	8	10	100
>74	93	2	4	7	100
Unknown	64	10	26	36	100
Total	74	4	22	26	100

As the chart shows, drivers with a BAC of .08 or higher were involved in more fatal car and motorcycle crashes than those with a BAC of .01 to .07.

Source: Traffic Safety Facts, 2007. National Highway Traffic Safety Administration, 2008.

Knowing Your BACs—Blood alcohol concentrations
The National Traffic Highway Safety Administration maintains data on alcohol-related car accident deaths in its Fatality Analysis Reporting System (FARS).

The amount of alcohol in your system is determined by measuring your BAC, or blood alcohol concentration, usually with a device called a breathalyzer. This test shows the ratio of alcohol to blood in your system and is expressed as a percentage.

A BAC reading of .10 means that alcohol makes up one-tenth of 1 percent of your blood. Young drivers show measurable driving

DID YOU KNOW?

Leading Causes of Death for People Ages 15–19

Rank	Cause	Percent of Deaths
1	Accidents (including car accidents)	49.8%
2	Homicide	14.1%
3	Suicide	12.4%
4	Cancer	5.3%
5	Heart Disease	2.7%

Accidents, homicides, and suicides are the three leading causes of death for teens ages 15–19. Alcohol use increases the odds of dying for each of these causes.

National Vital Statistics Report, November 2007.

impairment with BACs as low as .03 and significant impairment with BACS just under .10.

Younger drivers are high-risk drivers

Younger drivers are twice as likely as adults to be in a fatal car crash. The younger you are, the greater your chances of being in a serious accident. According to the Department of Transportation's Fatality Analysis Reporting System, 16-year-old drivers have crash rates three times greater than 17-year-olds and five times higher than 18-year-olds. In fact, car crashes are the number-one cause of death among all young people between the ages of 15 and 20.

Many reasons account for these alarming statistics about teen drivers: inexperience on the road; inadequate driving skills; poor judgment and decision making; too much night-time and weekend driving (when the chances of a car crash are greater); and impulsive, risk-taking behaviors such as speeding and drinking and driving.

How drinking affects driving

Drinking goes to your head; in other words, it has a profound effect on your brain. Specifically, it affects a part of the brain called the frontal lobe, which helps you think clearly, assess situations calmly, and make rational judgments. The frontal lobe also keeps you from making really bad, impulsive decisions.

Your frontal lobe is your best friend when you are driving—but only if you do not add alcohol to the mix. Even one drink impacts how the frontal lobe functions, along with how well you think, feel, and react in a stressful situation. And driving, which involves so many quick decisions, can be extremely stressful.

Driving requires multitasking

If you play soccer, football, or basketball, you know what multitasking is. You have to control both the ball and your body while you are constantly moving. You have to keep tabs on your teammates and watch out for your opponents. You have to follow the rules of the game, plus keep your eye on the field, on the ball, and on the goal or net. Multitasking takes a clear head and a lot of practice.

Driving requires multitasking too. You need to visually track several different moving objects at the same time, you need good hand-eye coordination, and you need to perform multiple tasks—all while you maintain control of your car and obey the laws.

TEENS SPEAK

"It Was Only Lemonade . . . "

Jason and I didn't really think any harm could come from a simple celebration. We were at my house, enjoying the first weekend of summer vacation and celebrating that we were officially juniors. We each had two hard lemonades each (that's lemonade made with alcohol).

It didn't seem like I drank much at all. In fact, it was so sweet that I couldn't even taste the alcohol. Later, someone told me there's more alcohol in this hard lemonade—5.2 percent in a 12-ounce can—than there is in many beers.

Neither one of us looked drunk when I asked to borrow my dad's car. He gave me the keys with a warning to stay close to home. Instead, we headed for the Parkstone Skyway; it's a mile-long suspension bridge that connects our island with the mainland.

Halfway across the bridge, something totally unexpected happened. A front tire blew on the car. I totally panicked! I felt so fuzzy-headed, I guess because of the lemonade, that I couldn't remember anything I learned in Driver's Ed about controlling the car. I hit the brakes hard, and then the car went into a spin, smashed into another car, and hit the guardrail on the side of the bridge. The car stopped, but I was so scared. What if someone was hurt? Fortunately, no one was seriously hurt, but my dad's car was totaled. And I got grounded from driving for my entire junior year!

When you drink, those abilities are impaired. You tend to focus your eyes on one area only, and you lose most of your peripheral vision. Your hand-eye coordination slows down, and you cannot handle the wheel or clutch and stick shift as well as usual. Your reaction times are off, and you brake too quickly or too slowly. You find it difficult to pay attention to more than one thing at a time, such as reading road signs and traffic signals, staying in your lane, following the speed limit, and watching out for pedestrians. When a person drinks and drives, all the talents that make someone a good and safe driver, and a responsible adult, are diminished—or disappear completely.

How much alcohol is too much?

Today all 50 states have BAC limits of .08 percent. That is two drinks or fewer in the first hour that someone may be drinking and one drink in each additional hour. These limits, of course, apply to *adult* drivers.

Fact Or Fiction?

> *"I never drink hard liquor like my parents do. I only drink beer. When I go to parties, I'll have just a couple of beers. I'm okay to drive, right?"*

The Facts: No, it's not all right to drive! One 12-ounce can of beer, one 5-ounce glass of wine, and 1 ¼ ounces of 80-proof hard liquor (the amount in a single drink) all have the *same* effect. Just one beer can affect how you drive. Your reaction time, judgment, and ability to think clearly are impaired. Two beers may put you over the legal BAC limit of .00—.02 percent for someone under the age of 21 and make you a candidate for either a serious accident or a DUI (driving under the influence) arrest.

Q & A

Question: I just got my intermediate license after having my permit and practicing my driving for six months—and I'm still not allowed to drive after 11:00 P.M., when the roads are practically empty! Why not?

Answer: Although the roads are less congested late at night, many of the drivers who are out there have been drinking far too much. How much? The rate of alcohol-involved fatal car crashes is more than three times greater at night (63 percent) than it is during daylight hours (19 percent). For all alcohol-involved crashes, the rate is five times higher at night than during the day. With those statistics (taken from a 2001 report of the National Highway Safety Bureau), you need a bit more time learning how to become a defensive driver before hitting the highway at night.

ZERO TOLERANCE LAWS EQUAL "ZERO" ALCOHOL

Experts have proven again and again that it takes much less alcohol to "influence" a teenager's driving. As a result, *all 50 states and the District of Columbia have zero tolerance laws for drivers under the age of 21*. That means if you are in that age group, it is illegal for you to operate a motor vehicle with *any* measurable amount of alcohol in your system, regardless of your state's BAC law for drivers over 21.

In other words, if you have one beer over the course of an evening and then drive–and you are caught–you may face the same DUI penalties that an older driver would, even if he or she drank *several* drinks. That is another powerful incentive not to drink and drive.

The BAC limits assigned to young drivers under the zero tolerance law vary by state and range from a BAC limit of .02 (the equivalent of one drink or less in an hour) to a BAC of 0.0, which means *no alcohol at all.* The BAC of 0.0 adheres to the letter of the law, since people under the age of 21 are not supposed to be drinking at all!

Knowing the laws and penalties for DUI

Educate yourself about your state's BAC limits and DUI penalties for adult drivers. If you are cited for DUI, many of these same penalties may apply to you. They may be even tougher–depending on your circumstances–and can include vehicle impoundment (taking and holding a person's vehicle until a fine is paid), vehicle confiscation, (process of legally taking a vehicle), or vehicle forfeiture (taking away a person's ownership of a vehicle); special license plates or plate markings; and ignition interlock (a device installed in your car that measures the alcohol in your breath before you can start the car).

Some eye-opening facts

You may find these facts about drinking to be surprising.

- The minimum drinking age in every state is 21. Yet, according to the Substance Abuse and Mental Health Services Administration (SAMHSA), 17 percent of people between ages 16 and 21 admitted to driving under the influence of alcohol.

- SAMHSA also reports that 4 percent of people who had reported driving under the influence were arrested and booked for DUI in the past year.

- According to the CDC, 19 percent of drivers ages 16 to 20 who died in a motor vehicle accident had been drinking alcohol.

- The CDC also reports that, in 2006, 13,470 people died in alcohol-impaired driving crashes. This accounted for 32 percent of all traffic-related deaths in the United States.

ROAD RAGE AND ALCOHOL USE

Road rage refers to a driver's overreaction to aggressive driving by another driver by retaliating with a violent act, usually an assault with a vehicle. This growing problem on the nation's roads is one that some people compare in its seriousness to drunk driving.

Alcohol, which intensifies feelings, is a major factor in many road rage incidents. Staying alcohol-free and following the rules of the road helps you avoid road rage incidents. Also remember to always wear your seat belt: It's the single greatest protection against road ragers and drunk drivers alike.

HELPING YOUNG DRIVERS
BECOME GOOD DRIVERS

Several years ago, traffic safety experts decided to address the problem of high-risk young drivers by introducing a driver education program that extended the learning process for teenage drivers. This program is called Graduated Driver Licensing (GDL). If your state does not have a GDL program now, it will certainly have one very soon.

All 50 states plus the District of Columbia have some type of GDL program in place.

While state GDL programs help new young drivers become skillful and responsible motorists, **Mothers Against Drunk Driving (MADD)** works tirelessly to keep young drivers safe and sober. Take a look at both programs now.

Major components of the GDL program

There are many steps on the way to getting your license.

Stage 1: Learner's Permit

- Be state's minimum age for a permit.
- Pass vision and knowledge tests and complete basic driver's education training.
- Travel with a licensed adult over the age of 21 at all times.
- Limit your number of teenage passengers.
- Observe zero alcohol law while driving.
- Remain free of crashes and convictions for at least six months.

Stage 2: Intermediate Provisional

- Complete Stage 1.
- Be your state's minimum age for an intermediate license.
- Pass road test and complete advanced driver's education training.
- Observe night-time driving restrictions (for example, no driving after 11:00 P.M.; travel with a licensed adult during late-night hours).
- Limit your number of teenage passengers.
- Observe zero alcohol law while driving.
- Remain accident- and conviction-free for at least 12-months.

Stage 3: Full Licensure

- Complete Stage 2.
- Be state's minimum age for full licensure.
- Observe zero-alcohol law while driving.

Young drivers must demonstrate responsible driving at each level—each having specific requirements and restrictions—before moving on to the next one.

MOTHERS AGAINST DRUNK DRIVING (MADD)

In 1980, Candace Lightner's 13-year-old daughter, Cari, was killed by a drunk driver who had just been released from jail two days before for another drunk driving offense—and he was still carrying a valid California driver's license.

Angered by the injustice of the situation, and fueled by grief, Candace Lightner met with a few friends to discuss what they could do to stop drunk drivers. MADD was born, and the rest is history. More than 20 years later, more than 600 MADD chapters exist in all 50 states, as well as in Canada, Guam, and Puerto Rico.

MADD's advocacy and activism efforts have resulted in thousands of federal and state anti-drunk driving laws. Among MADD's most significant accomplishments are:

- Introducing the "designated driver" program
- Establishing a Victim Bill of Rights
- Increasing the legal drinking age to 21 in all states
- Instituting tougher DUI penalties, including license revocation
- Advocating for a maximum BAC limit of .08 nationwide
- Championing zero tolerance laws for underage drivers

MADD is unquestionably the greatest advocacy and educational organization promoting safe, sober driving. Its mission statement is simple and clear: "To stop drunk driving, support victims of this violent crime, and prevent underage drinking."

SAYING NO TO DRINKING AND DRIVING

Choosing to say no is a tough decision, and only you can make it. By taking over the driver's seat, you are accepting one of the biggest responsibilities of being an adult: You are responsible for the lives of your passengers, yourself, and the other drivers on the road. Consider the consequences, in the short-term and in the long run.

Is the trade-off for making a bad decision worth it? How much do you value your life, and the lives of other people in your car and in other cars on the road? If you are having trouble making the right decision, remember that help is available. Talk to a friend, a counselor, your coach, or a teacher you trust.

If you are ever stuck in a situation where you are the driver but you've been drinking or you have to ride with someone who has been drinking, don't hesitate to call an adult (even your parents!) for help. Although you may worry that your parents will be angry, they would rather have you call for help than put yourself in a risky situation. You do not have to go it alone.

See also: Choices, Responsible; Effects on the Body; Ethnicity and Alcohol, Law and Drinking, The

FURTHER READING
Cefrey, Holly. *Frequently Asked Questions about Drinking and Driving.* New York: Rosen Publishing, 2008.
Grosshandler, Janet. *Coping with Drinking and Driving.* New York: Rosen Publishing Group, 1997.

■ DRINKING AND DRUGS

Remember those old horror pictures on late-night TV, where a mad scientist pours two chemicals together into a flask? Suddenly the liquid changes color, bubbles up, and overflows the rim in an explosion of steam and smoke.

An increasing number of Americans are performing a similar experiment—by mixing alcohol and other powerful drugs in their own bodies. **Drug interactions** (the effects that each drug has on the other) can be very dangerous. Even worse, the results are often as unpredictable as science fiction. You cannot be sure what will happen each time you try another test, or repeat the same test one more time.

In real life, the experimenters often wind up in the hospital or in other health-care facilities. The Substance Abuse and Mental Health Services Administration estimates that in 2006, 2.5 million people between the ages of 12 and 17 received substance abuse treatment. Approximately 731,000 received treatment for alcohol abuse, which is 34 percent of all those receiving substance abuse treatment.

Treatment professionals have long noted the obvious similarities between alcohol **abuse** and drug addiction as individual behaviors.

Eventually they coined the term *substance abuse* to cover all types of chemical misuse and dependence, whether that involves alcohol, illegal drugs, prescription drugs, natural or artificial chemicals, or any combination thereof.

Unfortunately, some teenagers too have fallen victim to multiple substance abuse behaviors. Over the years, as both alcohol and illicit drug use has become more widespread among young people, many of them have been combining the two.

In fact, most teenagers who consume heavy quantities of alcohol also use illicit drugs. The National Household Survey on Drug Abuse issued some startling numbers for the year 2000. Some 66 percent of 12- to 17-year-old heavy drinkers (meaning, they drank five or more alcoholic drinks on one occasion, on at least five different occasions that month) also used illicit drugs. More than 40 percent of binge drinkers (they drank five or more drinks on one occasion, less than five times that month) did the same.

Even some moderate drinkers who never binged used drugs, but not quite as many as heavier drinkers—about 20 percent. The only 12 to 17-year-olds who seemed to avoid drugs were those who abstained from alcohol as well. Only 4 percent of kids who did not drink at all (in the month prior to the survey) used illicit drugs. Fortunately for the health of American kids, that was still the solid majority of the population—83 percent of 12 to 17-year-olds, according to the Household Survey.

Statistics such as these can be very convincing. They show a connection between alcohol abuse and the use of illicit drugs. Does one behavior cause the other?

WHAT ARE THE LINKS?

The Household Survey figures seem to indicate that the more a teenager drinks, the more likely he or she is to use illicit drugs as well. Other surveys show that most kids who use illicit drugs experimented with alcohol first.

Stepping-stones and gateways

In the past, researchers believed that some drugs were "stepping-stones" to others. They believed that a person who drank alcohol would sometimes move on to other, usually illegal drugs and leave behind their drinking.

But more recent behavior patterns have led many of the experts to replace the stepping-stone comparison with another one: They call

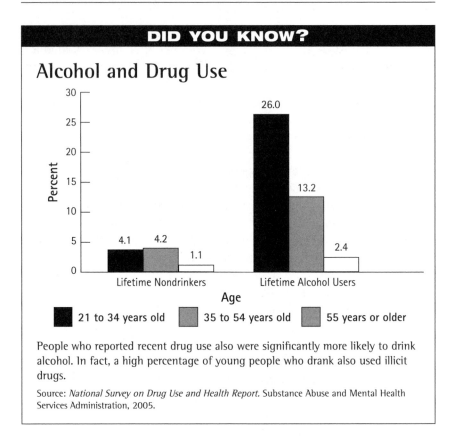

DID YOU KNOW?

Alcohol and Drug Use

People who reported recent drug use also were significantly more likely to drink alcohol. In fact, a high percentage of young people who drank also used illicit drugs.

Source: *National Survey on Drug Use and Health Report.* Substance Abuse and Mental Health Services Administration, 2005.

alcohol one of the **gateway drugs,** along with **nicotine** (the addictive chemical in tobacco) and marijuana.

These researchers do not claim that *everyone* who drinks tries drugs; many go no further, and may even stop drinking. But they have identified a path that most teenage drug users follow, starting with cigarettes and alcohol, then adding marijuana, and continuing to other common illicit drugs. For boys, the most common gateway is alcohol; for girls it is alcohol combined with cigarettes. Almost no teenagers use illicit drugs without first passing through these gateways.

Some experts in the field are uneasy with the term "gateway." First of all, they say, there is no evidence that alcohol use actually *causes* kids to try other drugs. It may be that the same reasons that cause some kids to abuse alcohol also lead them to use illicit drugs. The experts also fear that the public may forget that tobacco and alcohol

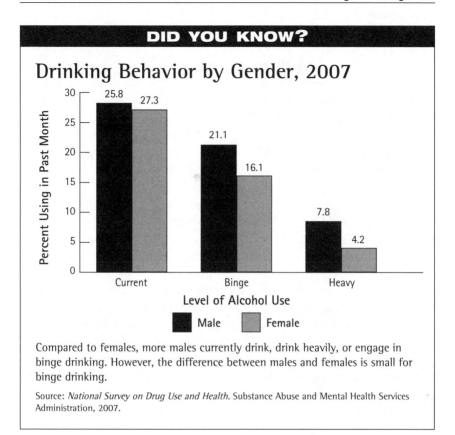

DID YOU KNOW?

Drinking Behavior by Gender, 2007

Compared to females, more males currently drink, drink heavily, or engage in binge drinking. However, the difference between males and females is small for binge drinking.

Source: *National Survey on Drug Use and Health.* Substance Abuse and Mental Health Services Administration, 2007.

alone harm far more people than illicit drugs, which most Americans still avoid.

Some of these researchers prefer the term *markers.* They say that alcohol and cigarettes are markers, or warning signs, that a teenager is at high risk for using other drugs as well. Using that terminology, the strongest marker of all is *early* drinking. Two-thirds of all those who start drinking before age 16 eventually use illicit drugs, while only one-fourth of those who wait until they are 17 to drink do so.

Reinforcement and cross-tolerance

Many kids who abuse alcohol may have emotional problems that make them likely candidates for drug abuse. Other kids may use drugs simply because they are available. But are there more specific links between the two behaviors? Are there ways in which alcohol directly influences a kid to use another drug?

One obvious factor is that anyone who drinks to the point of intoxication does not have the same good judgment he or she has while sober. If you were a young drug dealer trying to win a new customer, you could hardly find a more gullible candidate than a drunk. Even kids who know the facts about drug interactions, and who have no desire to pick up an expensive and troublesome habit, may put all those doubts aside while under the influence of alcohol.

Even if one drug does not actually lead a user to try another drug, once he or she does try it, the two behaviors often reinforce each other. For example, drinkers who have been introduced to marijuana may later use it in the hope that it may alleviate the miseries of a hangover. People who use **amphetamine,** a drug that can make their minds feel overactive or wired-up, may then drink alcohol just to calm down or fall asleep. Also, alcohol abusers may use amphetamines to wake themselves up after drinking too much. They are fooling themselves—they may feel awake, but their coordination remains unreliable and they should never attempt to drive in that state.

People who use more than one drug can develop **cross-tolerance** and **cross-addiction.** Heavy drinkers usually develop a **tolerance** to alcohol, needing to drink more to feel the same effect. Often, they become tolerant to other drugs too, even before they try them. Doctors often give higher doses of anesthetics (painkillers) to surgery patients who are alcoholic; a normal dose does not do the job. Alcohol abusers who "medicate themselves" with illicit drugs do the same—they need to take more of the drug to feel any effect.

In cross-addiction, people may use a substitute drug if their primary drug is not readily available. For example, heroin addicts frequently drink alcohol to relieve withdrawal symptoms when they cannot obtain any heroin.

Sadly, some doctors prescribe sedatives to certain patients troubled by anxiety and sleeplessness without knowing that the symptoms were caused by the early stages of alcoholism. Their patients often develop cross-addiction to alcohol *and* the sedative.

Researchers also suspect that a physical interaction between alcohol and certain drugs strengthens cross-addiction. Heavy drinkers who abuse heroin or barbiturates can sometimes slide into full **dependency** (alcoholism) in much less time than it takes someone who sticks to alcohol alone.

Alcohol and tobacco

The drug that seems to go "best" with alcohol is **nicotine**, the chemical that makes cigarettes so addictive. People who drink heavily almost always smoke cigarettes too. According to a 1998 report of the National Institute on Alcohol Abuse and Alcoholism, "Extensive research supports the popular observation that 'smokers drink and drinkers smoke.'"

The research from over a decade ago still holds true today. According to the 2007 National Survey on Drug Use and Health, 58.1 percent of heavy alcohol users also admitted to smoking in the past month. This compares to only 16.4 percent of nondrinkers who admitted to smoking in the past month. Forty-five percent of current smokers admitted to binge drinking the prior month.

Cigarettes are not illegal or illicit, at least for adults. However, they are one of the most addictive drugs on the market, as millions of people can tell you from bitter experience. And while the short-term risks of smoking are small compared with alcohol and illicit drugs (for example, you aren't as likely to have a car accident when smoking as you are when drinking), the long-term damage makes cigarettes one of the most harmful drugs of all. Smoking tobacco can cause lung and other cancers, emphysema, severe heart and circulation disease, blindness, and a host of other problems.

TEENS SPEAK

Which Is Worse: Alcohol or Tobacco?

"People can sometimes be too smart for their own good," said Sorosh, a 14-year-old boy who lives in California. "Like, for example, my older sister."

Sorosh's family emigrated from Iran just after he was born. His parents honored the Muslim prohibition against alcohol and tried to get their children to do the same. "But ever since my sister started college, she hangs around with these kids who drink pitchers of beer every Friday and Saturday night," Sorosh said. "When my parents tried to argue with her, she just turned it around and talked about my father's smoking.

"She used to say that smoking was much worse than drinking. That's a big issue in my house, because my father smokes at least a pack a day, and we are always trying to get him to give it up. My sister would bring home booklets she got in school about the harmful effects of tobacco.

"As long as Dad smokes, she won't let him give her any advice. But in the end, the joke's on her: Since she's been drinking she started smoking too, just like all her friends who drink. They light up as soon as they get together and keep smoking all night.

"My sister still drinks beer on the weekends, but now she smokes every day too. My father has finally signed up for an antismoking program in order to get my sister to stop too.

"Now she listens to them a little more. Lately she's even skipped going out on a few Saturday nights."

EATING BEHAVIORS

Alcohol abuse is also often connected with another serious problem—eating disorders. Drinking can complicate and exacerbate **anorexia nervosa** and **bulimia**, which together affect several million Americans.

People with anorexia nervosa are unwilling or unable to eat the minimum amount of food necessary to stay alive and healthy. They usually suffer from the mistaken idea that their bodies are unattractively fat. Bulimia sufferers also are obsessed with their weight. They eat normally much of the time, but they are subject to cycles of binge eating followed by vomiting or other extreme measures to get rid of the excess food. The large majority of patients are women; often the problem first appears in the teenage years.

A large proportion of eating disorder patients, perhaps a third, are also alcoholics, and many abuse other substances as well. Researchers have not established a direct link between the two behaviors, according to a 2002 NIAAA report entitled "Eating Disorders and Alcohol Use Disorders."

HOW DRUGS INTERACT

In recent years, television dramas have given the public a new respect for the doctors and nurses who staff hospital emergency rooms. One of the most difficult tasks these overworked professionals face is diagnosis: Why has this man stopped breathing? Why does that woman have a dangerously rapid heartbeat?

Drug interactions are one of the most difficult diagnoses to call, mostly because they are so complicated. For example, low amounts of alcohol cause a very different reaction to many drugs than large amounts, while alcoholics (even if they have not had a drink that day) may react in yet another way. A person's age, weight, and sex can also play a part, as can the amount of food a person ate before or while he or she was using drugs.

Some drug combinations can have a reinforcing effect. Two depressants taken at the same time may make people so mellow that they pass out or even stop breathing.

Q & A

Question: What happens when people mix alcohol and ecstasy?

Answer: Ecstasy, or E, is a synthetic "club drug" that is somewhat similar to methamphetamine. Alcohol and ecstasy both dehydrate (remove water from) the body, and both can cause a rise in body temperature. When you add the two together, you may cause heat stroke and can damage your liver and kidney. If that isn't enough damage, people report that the combination makes for a severe "come down."

Other drug duos can cancel out each other, at least in terms of behavior: A depressant can bring a person down from a high so he or she appears almost normal. But beware: The same two drugs may reinforce each other internally, causing harm to the body. A few of the possible negative interactions with alcohol that doctors and ER staff have seen are

- Amphetamines: can cause severe gastrointestinal distress (stomach and intestinal problems); can lead to an alcohol overdose, since the amphetamine will prevent a drinker from passing out
- Barbiturates: can cause death from a reinforced effect on the heart or lungs
- Codeine: respiratory arrest (you stop breathing)
- Darvon: cardiac arrest (your heart stops working)
- Heroin (or any injected drug): high risk of liver damage

- Marijuana: greater effect on coordination and mental skills than either one by itself

- Tranquilizers: can lead to suicide or vehicle crashes, since coordination and common sense are at a low, even though the user may not *feel* all that drunk

Fact Or Fiction?

Inhalants aren't really so dangerous; otherwise, they wouldn't be sold.

The Facts: Inhalants *are* dangerous! Cars are dangerous when misused, and they're sold too. The fact is, various fluids, sprays, and gases that kids often use to get high can have serious effects. Whether kids use them repeatedly at one time, or frequently over time, they can lead to brain damage and even death—especially when combined with alcohol.

MOOD SWINGS

Therapists who treat mental disease estimate that 2 million Americans suffer from **bipolar disorder**, also called manic-depressive disorder. Even without touching a drug or medication, they swing between moods of mania, when they feel full of energy and confidence, and moods of deep depression or sadness. Often an incapacitating illness preventing the patient from performing the ordinary tasks of daily life, bipolar disorder is difficult for doctors to treat.

Ups and downs

People with bipolar disorder are in danger of becoming addicted to legal and illegal drugs. Even when not actually bipolar (and most people are not), individuals can still experience that kind of emotional roller-coaster if they abuse more than one drug. In many cases, alcohol and drug abusers can develop a pattern of behavior that is just as incapacitating, and just as difficult to treat.

Many drugs, including alcohol, barbiturates, and sedatives (such as Valium) are depressants. When their full effects kick in, people are less alert and may nod off. Other drugs are stimulants, such as cocaine, amphetamines, and Ritalin; under their influence, people feel wide awake and full of energy.

When people use illicit drugs, in a way they are "writing their own prescriptions." However, they can't usually control the dose very well. When they feel too manic, they may take a dose of alcohol to calm down or fall asleep. When they are too drowsy, they make take a dose of stimulant to keep them awake or to keep from feeling depressed. Before long, they are suffering the same effects as true bipolar patients. It can be difficult to climb out of this trap.

The mood swing of addiction

People can experience another kind of "mood swing" as they develop a dependency or addiction to one or more drugs. Therapists describe the four stages that teenagers go through as they experiment with a new drug:

1. Learning the mood swing. This is when teens first experience the mood change that comes with drug use. They may try to repeat that feeling through occasional drug use.

2. Seeking the mood swing. In this stage kids use the drug or drugs more to avoid negative feelings and stress than to experience the "good" mood.

3. Preoccupation with the mood swing. The need to change their mood becomes the main focus of the drug abusers' lives.

4. Using drugs to feel normal. The drug may lose its ability to make abusers feel better. It just holds off the bad feelings, which now include guilt and shame over being addicted, pressure to raise money to buy the drug or drugs, fear of being caught, and the painful symptoms of **withdrawal**.

COUNSELING, REHABILITATION, AND ABSTINENCE

In recent years, the treatment community has become more skillful in diagnosing and treating people who abuse more than one drug. Counselors are trained to inquire about or seek evidence for cross-addiction, and most treatment programs and centers are set up to deal with the problem.

For the most part, therapists treat cross-addicted individuals the same way they treat those dependent on alcohol alone. Patients need to address the reasons for their harmful behaviors, and they need to develop healthier social and behavior patterns to keep them from reverting to drug abuse.

The main impact is on the medical aspect of treatment, including **detoxification** (cleansing the body of the effects of addiction) and any medicines used in treatment. People seeking treatment must be totally honest with therapists in order to allow them to devise the best and safest methods to treat each individual patient.

BAD COMBINATION

Both alcohol and illicit drugs can be difficult to handle and very dangerous. Combined, as they often are, they present a major challenge to physical and mental health that many people fail to overcome.

See also: Effects on the Body; Recovery and Treatment, Tolerance and Reverse Tolerance

FURTHER READING

Carson-DeWitt, Rosalyn, et al. *Drugs, Alcohol, and Tobacco: Learning About Addictive Behavior.* New York: Macmillan Reference USA, 2003.

Lohman, Jessica. *The Truth About Drugs and Teens: An Informed Perspective.* Bloomington, Ind.: AuthorHouse, 2005.

Seixas, Judith S., and Geraldine Youcha. *Drugs, Alcohol, and Your Children: What Every Parent Needs to Know.* New York: Penguin, 1999.

■ DRIVING WHILE INTOXICATED

See: Drinking and Driving

■ DRINKING ON COLLEGE CAMPUSES

The college experience does seem to lend itself to drinking. On the average, high school kids who are planning to attend college drink *less* than their fellow students. But once they get there, their behavior changes. College students drink *more* alcohol than those in their age group who do not attend college.

Years ago, college was an elite experience. Only a small number of kids whose families had the means to send them could hope to attend. An even smaller number managed to obtain scholarships through hard

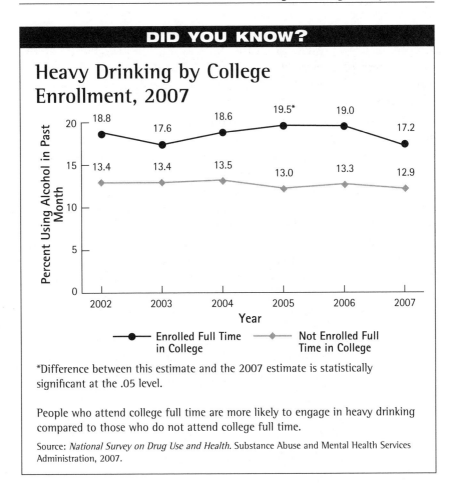

DID YOU KNOW?

Heavy Drinking by College Enrollment, 2007

*Difference between this estimate and the 2007 estimate is statistically significant at the .05 level.

People who attend college full time are more likely to engage in heavy drinking compared to those who do not attend college full time.

Source: *National Survey on Drug Use and Health.* Substance Abuse and Mental Health Services Administration, 2007.

work and luck. Today, the majority of kids in high school can expect to get some amount of higher education. Attending college has become part of the experience of growing up for the majority of American youth.

For the most part, college is a positive experience. Students gain the knowledge they need to succeed in the working world, and refine their social and intellectual skills so they can take full part in adult life.

For many students, one of these social achievements is learning how to drink sensibly. Unfortunately, some of their fellow students who drink fail that course. America's colleges are experiencing some serious problems with **alcohol abuse** among students.

If you are planning to attend college, try to familiarize yourself with these problems, so you are better prepared to handle them sensibly when the time comes.

WHAT ARE THE NUMBERS?

According to the results from the 2007 Monitoring the Future study, 66.6 percent of college students admitted to drinking in the past 30 days. Almost 47 percent stated they had been drunk, while 41 percent engaged in binge drinking. A 2005 study by the Core Institute of Southern Illinois University found that 72.8 percent of college students used alcohol in the past 30 days. The institute also found that 34.2 percent of college men were heavy and frequent drinkers, compared to 20.1 percent of college women.

The majority of college students manage to handle this culture without suffering any lasting damage to their physical or mental health. But not everyone is that fortunate.

According to a U.S. government Web site, "College Drinking Prevention," an estimated 31 percent of college students meet the criteria for alcohol abuse. Another 6 percent are considered to have a dependence on alcohol. The following is a list of alcohol-related consequences for college students between the ages of 18 and 24:

- Seventeen hundred students die every year from alcohol-related injuries, including car crashes.

- Some 2.1 million students drove under the influence of alcohol.

- Five hundred ninety-nine thousand students are injured while under the influence of alcohol.

- More than 696,000 students are assaulted by another student who has been drinking.

- Some 97,000 students are victims of date rape or sexual assault.

- Approximately 5 percent of students are involved with campus security or the police as a result of student drinking.

- One hundred ten thousand students are arrested for an alcohol-related violation, such as public drunkenness.

- More than 150,000 students develop an alcohol-related health problem.

CULTURAL ATTITUDES AND EXPERIMENTATION

For better or worse, alcohol is part of the traditional culture of most of America's colleges and universities. Long-established traditions of social drinking are passed down from older students to younger, through casual conversations, stories about the "good old days," dorm room parties, and socializing at off-campus bars and taverns.

These traditions were established in the days when most states allowed the sale of alcoholic beverages to 18-year-olds, exactly the age of most college freshmen. Going off to college and coming "of age" for drinking happened at the same time. The legal age has changed, but college life has not fully adjusted to the change in the laws. Needless to say, the many upperclassmen and graduate students who are 21 or over make it relatively easy for underage college kids to get access to alcoholic beverages.

New students find it difficult to resist these traditions, even if they are wary or skeptical. Most freshmen feel an exciting sense of freedom. Those whose parents had previously kept a close eye on their behavior now have to rely on their own sense of responsibility, which is not always up to the task.

College faculty members and administrators do not have the same role in monitoring student behavior as teachers and principals in public or private high school. Unlike the teachers whom freshmen may remember, college professors, lecturers, and teaching assistants feel no obligation to keep tabs on the on-campus behavior of their students, let alone their off-campus life. They are paid to teach particular skills or a specialized body of knowledge. They are not expected to help kids navigate the competing demands of college life.

Alcohol has always been part of the culture of fraternities and sororities. Drinking games, in which students (especially pledges trying to gain admission) drink dangerous quantities of alcohol in dangerously short periods of time, are notorious. At some fraternities in the past, no event was complete without a few beer kegs. Without empty bottles around, no one can keep track of how much anyone has drunk.

Fact Or Fiction?

The reason for heavy drinking in fraternities and sororities is that kids who like to drink are the ones who join in the first place.

The Facts: The association isn't true. Recent studies have shown that once fraternity and sorority members graduate and move on to new environments, their drinking declines to a level that is normal for their age and background. Researchers now suspect that "Greeks" (fraternity members) drink more while at college because that's the prevailing "culture" among their peers and not because of any particular "fraternity personality type."

Of course, not every student pledges a sorority or fraternity. However, alcohol has always been associated with many other sectors of college society as well, from jocks to student intellectuals to the faculty. With the exception of a handful of institutions founded or run by religious denominations, few institutions in American life have been more accepting of alcohol than colleges.

In a 2007 study in the *Journal of College Student Development,* the authors found that excessive drinking hurts academic performance. In this study, the authors discovered that students who engage in binge drinking had grades that are significantly lower than students who do not engage in this behavior. In a 2008 study in *Psychology of Addictive Behaviors,* researchers found that students who are heavy drinkers are at an increased risk of dropping out of college. The consequences of drinking are not just related to poor performance; they can ultimately influence whether or not someone stays in school.

In 1998, The NIAAA established a task force to investigate problems associated with college drinking and to recommend solutions. The task force concluded that the most important issue was the culture itself. No lasting change was possible if colleges focused only on the individual drinker.

College culture may be changing, however, at least as far as tolerating underage drinking and abusive drinking at parties. Some college administrations have tried to limit advertising and other alcohol promotions on campus. Others have encouraged alcohol-free dormitories and social clubs. Several college towns have introduced **tagging** of beer kegs, in which sellers must keep track of purchasers.

According to a 1998 story in *U.S. News and World Report,* about 30 percent of all colleges had instituted more restrictive drinking policies in the previous two years. In one popular measure, colleges decided to fine underage students for drinking and to fine of-age students for having more than a certain amount of alcohol in their dorm rooms.

Fraternities are also feeling some pressure to change due to some highly publicized incidents of fatal alcohol poisoning caused by overdrinking. Expensive increases in insurance premiums, to cover alcohol-related lawsuits, may also convince local and national fraternity financial officers. In 1997, the National Interfraternity Council recommended that member fraternities set up alcohol-free chapters. By 2001, two-thirds of all national fraternities had at least one such chapter, and eleven were working toward a complete alcohol-free policy.

These measures are having an impact. The Core Institute at Southern Illinois University reported in the late 1990s that binge drinking had declined by 13 percent on campuses since 1980. Other studies have even shown an increase in the number of students abstaining from alcohol completely.

However, more recent research indicates this trend has not been consistent. Authors of a 2009 study in the *Journal of Studies on Alcohol and Drugs* found that binge drinking increased between 1999 and 2005. The number of college students who admitted to binge drinking increased from 41.7 percent in 1999 and to 44.7 percent in 2005. The authors also found that more students were driving under the influence of alcohol.

A 2008 study in the *Journal of American College Health* indicates that exposing students to "social norms" can help reduce problem drinking. Students often overestimate the amount of drinking on college campuses. The authors of this study found that by publicizing survey results about alcohol use, as well as healthy behaviors, or social norms, problem drinking decreased. Some of them had previously believed that alcohol abuse was an *expected* part of college life. Conformity—doing what everyone else is doing—is sometimes hard to resist.

TEENS SPEAK

A Freshman Learns Fast

Sean, an 18-year-old college freshman, is living away from home for the first time. He still hangs out with a bunch of high school classmates who all picked the same state college campus.

"The first week of school, before regular classes started, we all went to a tavern just off campus to party. It was really crowded, so a couple of older guys didn't have too much trouble getting us in without getting carded. We weren't a big drinking crowd at Franklin, but somehow we felt that college was different. Like it was expected of us to get drunk. By midnight we were so boozed, we kind of staggered home.

"I had a roaring hangover the next day, but it was an exciting experience in a way. Like, now I'm one of the men. But then a couple of the guys started bringing six-packs into the dorm during the week, and we'd sit up drinking for hours. It was getting in the way of my studying, and frankly, I didn't enjoy it all that much.

"Then the college ran a student alcohol survey. I was averaging at least three beers a day, which I thought was more or less typical. But it turned out that only six percent of all undergraduates were drinking as much as me! I was trying to keep up, but with who?

"I was so happy to drop the mid-week drinking. I have more time to study, and to sleep, and even to get to know my new roommates. And I'm saving a few bucks too."

MONEY AND COLLEGE STUDENTS

College students as a rule have greater disposable income than their counterparts in high school. They are more likely to work (around 40 percent have jobs), and any money they receive from parents is likely to come in a larger sum.

In any case, inexpensive alcohol is readily available. Many off-campus bars provide low-cost promotions to attract students, including cheap or two-for-one beer nights. When allowed, they often advertise these specials on campus too.

The scholarly journal *Health and Place* reported on a 2003 study of eight campuses that measured the extent of heavy drinking (having five or more drinks on one occasion) against the density of alcohol outlets near the campus. As common sense suggests, there was a strong correlation between the density (number of outlets per square mile) and the amount of problem drinking.

For students at high-bar-density colleges, with competition driving down the price of a drink, heavy drinking may be the cheapest form of entertainment available. Two-for-one hours, cheap-beer Wednesdays, ladies' nights, and other promotions tend to perpetuate the culture of college drinking.

DRINKING AND RISKY SEX

Whatever you might think after watching TV shows about teenagers or hearing popular songs, many young people are not sexually experienced when they enter college. Almost 40 percent of 12th-grade students in the 2007 Youth Risk Behavior Survey (YRBS) had not had a single sexual partner (37.2 percent of boys and 33.8 percent of girls). Those who did engage in sex in high school generally had only one or two partners.

As teenagers become young adults, though, the situation changes. The respected *Morbidity and Mortality Weekly Report* of the Centers for Disease Control and Prevention reported in 1997 that 86 percent of college students had engaged in sexual intercourse at least once—and 68 percent within the three months before the survey.

These statistics sound bare and lifeless. After all, sexual feelings and behaviors involve so many complicated emotions—romantic love, the need for intimacy and affection, trust, fear, shame, and self-respect, to name just a few. Also, sexual behavior is influenced by powerful physical drives.

All in all, the factors that push people toward intimate relations with other people, or that hold them back, are often difficult to manage. As college students experiment with their newfound independence and freedom from supervision, some of them make errors of judgment. They may take chances they later regret, or find themselves engaging in activity they had meant to avoid.

Considering the risks involved, both physical and emotional, in being sexually active, doesn't it make sense to have a reasonably clear head when you decide when, where, and with whom to have sex?

Sexual behavior is considered risky if it puts either partner at risk of becoming infected with HIV (the AIDS virus) or any other STD (**sexually transmitted disease**), or if it can lead to an unwanted pregnancy. Examples of risky behavior are having sex with several different partners, having sex with a partner you don't know, having unprotected sex with a high-risk partner (such as someone who injects drugs with a needle), or having sex without using birth control. Every method of birth control carries its own level of risk; some can safely prevent pregnancy but do not protect against STDs. Without a condom, any sexual contact can be considered risky sex, outside of a monogamous marriage or similar relationship.

Risky sexual behavior is quite common on college campuses. As reported in a 2008 article in *Psychology and Health,* researchers found that alcohol use influences risky sexual behaviors. In this study, the authors found that alcohol intoxication influenced men's decision making regarding sexual behavior but not women's. Men are likely to engage in riskier behavior if they have consumed alcohol. A 2008 article in *AIDS Behavior* also found that drinking influences risky sexual behavior. The authors of this study reported that alcohol use increased the chances of women having unprotected sex with a steady partner. However, alcohol use by men did not influence the decision to use a condom.

A 2007 study in *Addictive Behaviors* reinforces the connection between alcohol use and risky sexual activity. The authors found that college students were more likely to have unprotected sex with a "non-steady" partner if they had been drinking. In a 2009 study, published in the *Journal of Studies on Alcohol and Drugs,* the authors discovered that women who regularly drink in bars are more likely to engage in sexual risk taking. However, in this study the risk taking was more likely to occur when a female was with a regular partner instead of someone new.

ATHLETICS AND DRINKING

In the minds of many college students, alcohol and athletics go hand in hand. After all, liquor companies sponsor collegiate athletic events; tailgate parties are notorious for consuming large amounts of beer; and college jocks have a reputation for drinking.

The notion may be a bit exaggerated, but not by much. According to the Core Institute of Southern Illinois University 1996 report, 88 percent of the athletes drink at least once a year, as compared with 82 percent of the general student population. But heavy drinking is more of a problem. According to college alcohol expert Henry Wechsler, more than half of male athletes, and close to half of the female athletes, engage in binge drinking.

In recent years, college athletic departments have instituted major antialcohol and antidrug programs. They are trying to break the connection, real or perceived, between sports and alcohol.

In 2001, the National Collegiate Athletic Association (NCAA) surveyed its member institutions about their alcohol policies and programs. More than 500 schools replied, and the results seemed encouraging. Sixty-six percent had instituted alcohol and drug education programs for athletes and 26 percent for staff. Nearly half had mandatory random drug and alcohol tests; athletes testing positive faced suspension or removal from their teams.

The same survey showed some improvement in the advertising situation as well. Eighty-two percent of the colleges reported that they did not allow alcohol ads on sports arena signs, and 77 percent kept them out of their game programs.

Q & A

Question: If college athletes drink more heavily than non-athletes, is that true for high school athletes too?

Answer: Not necessarily. In fact, an Indiana University study of 69,000 students in grades 7–12 in that state found that kids who participated in at least one team sport used alcohol at about the same rate as those who did not participate. However, the athletes were less likely to smoke cigarettes or use marijuana.

ALCOHOL AND SEXUAL VIOLENCE

Sexual violence takes place when one person forces another person to engage in sexual activity. Nearly all the victims are women.

Many types of sexual violence are no more common at colleges than anywhere else. But acquaintance rape and date rape have become a major concern in recent years on campuses across the United States. In the vast majority of rapes committed on college campuses (more than eight out of 10), the attacker is someone the victim knows—an acquaintance. In most cases, the crime occurs in a social setting, usually on a date.

A January 2001 Department of Justice report, *The Sexual Victimization of College Women,* reported that some 3 percent of college women are victims of rape or attempted rape each year. About 13 percent report being stalked.

Alcohol and, to a lesser extent, other drugs play a huge role in acquaintance rape. In the large majority of reported rape cases on college campuses, both those who commit the assault and their victims were drinking. Alcohol tends to cause aggressive behavior by an attacker and weakens a victim's defenses. With acquaintance rape, other aspects of alcohol come into play as well.

Most men know it's wrong to force their sexual attention on an unwilling partner. With some men, though, alcohol lowers their moral inhibitions; or they may excuse their behavior even while it is taking place by saying, "The drink made me do it." They also may associate alcohol with sex, feel more sexually aroused when drinking, and make the false assumption that any woman who drinks is always receptive to sexual advances. Sexual signals between men and women can be subtle and easy to misinterpret. If some men always think they are desired, they surely believe so under the influence.

When the woman is drinking, the risk of sexual assault increases. If a man and a woman drink the same quantity of alcohol, the woman is more likely to be intoxicated, due to differences in the way their bodies process alcohol. This puts a woman at a severe physical disadvantage if she tries to resist a sexual advance. It also weakens her decision-making ability, making her more likely to get into dangerous situations and less able to figure out how to escape.

As if alcohol isn't dangerous enough, drugs sometimes enter the picture as well. Some "club drugs," secretly dropped into a woman's drink, may make her unable to move or cause her to lose consciousness.

As colleges have become aware of this situation, most of them have begun serious education campaigns and have imposed more serious penalties on violators—a trend that is likely to continue.

Whatever policies college administrations may adopt, the practical responsibility rests with the individual. Female students must be aware of these risks before and during dates, even with guys they know. Male students should take a good look at their behavior, in advance and after the fact. They must learn not to use alcohol as an excuse for actions that may lead to suspension or expulsion from college, criminal prosecution, or jail. Also, they should face up to and reject any behavior that dishonors them and the values they uphold.

ALCOHOL AND CHUGGING: SUDDEN DEATH

Every now and then, an isolated incident can break into national news coverage and spark a debate on issues that previously had been ignored. That happened in August 1997, after an incident at Louisiana State University in Baton Rouge.

A group of fraternity pledges went with their frat brothers to a nearby bar, where they drank a concoction of rum, whiskey, and liqueur. They eventually had to be carried out and driven home. When the campus police arrived at the frat house, they found more than 20 young men passed out. Four were taken to the hospital, where one of them, with an astonishing **blood alcohol level** (BAL) of .588, died of alcohol poisoning. Just one month later, a freshman at the Massachusetts Institute of Technology went into a coma at a fraternity party when his BAL reached .41. He died three days later.

Chugging, the practice of drinking alcohol faster than the body can handle, is believed to be relatively common at colleges. Chugging can take many forms. On college campuses, it is often associated with drinking games, involving swigging contests, spiked Jell-O cubes, and other ways of getting alcohol down the hatch as fast as possible. Often, some form of chugging is part of the hazing of pledges, which still takes place at some fraternities. In hazing, candidates for admission to a fraternity have to perform unpleasant, humiliating, and/or dangerous tasks as part of the initiation process.

Chugging is a potentially deadly practice. Even the most neutral and nonjudgmental experts, who may disagree about whether alcohol is a boon or a poison, offer the same warning about chugging–don't do it.

KIDS OR ADULTS?

College is the first phase of adult life for countless American teens, a time when they can make lifestyle choices independent of parental control. It is also a time when they must pay the full consequences of bad or uninformed decisions. If they are smart, they will come to college already prepared with information and sensible ideas to help them face the challenges of alcohol as mature young adults.

See also: Alcohol Abuse, The Risks of; Alcohol and Violence; Alcohol Poisoning; Tolerance and Reverse Tolerance

FURTHER READING
Dowdall, George W. *College Drinking: Reframing a Social Problem.* Westport, Conn.: Praeger Publishers, 2008.

Nuwer, Hank. *Wrongs of Passage: Fraternities, Sororities, Hazing, and Binge Drinking.* Bloomington: Indiana University Press, 1999.

Salz, Robert F., and William DeJong. *Reducing Alcohol Problems on Campus: A Guide to Planning and Evaluation.* Washington, D.C.: National Institutes of Health, 2002.

Walters, Scott. T., and John S. Baer. *Talking With College Students About Alcohol: Motivational Strategies for Reducing Abuse.* New York: The Guilford Press, 2005.

■ DRUG ABUSE AND ALCOHOL
See: Drinking and Drugs; Drinking on College Campuses

■ EFFECTS OF ALCOHOL ON THE BODY
The body can handle modest amounts of alcohol, though the amount varies with age, gender, and size. It requires a delicate balance. Take in too much, too quickly, and a lot of systems go seriously out of whack.

Think of your body as a complex, almost miraculous machine. It can run like clockwork by itself, and even accomplish great feats—but only if you treat it with care.

METABOLISM
The process of **metabolism,** or breaking down what your body takes in, works like this: first, alcohol is absorbed into your bloodstream through the different parts of the digestive system—the mouth, stomach, and intestines. Then, your liver metabolizes the alcohol into products your body can handle better. Finally, some of these products get used or misused in the body while the others are eliminated as waste.

All along this path, alcohol interacts with the other foods and drugs it finds in your system. And it leaves its effects, visible and invisible, on the body.

Absorption
Each time you drink, the alcohol in the beverage starts to work almost instantly. Before you can even swallow, some of it gets absorbed into the blood through the mucus membranes of the mouth. But 95 percent does manage to slither down to the stomach. The stomach, in turn, allows 25 percent to pass through its lining into the blood and pushes the rest into the intestine. That remaining 70 percent is gradually absorbed through the walls of the intestines.

A little bit of the alcohol evaporates out of the blood as it passes through the lungs. The lungs in turn exhale the alcohol into the air. Other tiny quantities evaporate through the skin.

When a person has one standard-sized drink on an empty stomach, with no other digestion work to do, the efficient gastrointestinal tract (digestive system) can complete the absorption process in 30 minutes.

But that is like running an assembly line so fast that the parts pile up dangerously in front of the next guy on the line—the liver. He just can't handle the volume.

A full stomach usually cuts the absorption rate in half so that the bloodstream has an hour to absorb the drink. Foods with high fat content are especially good at slowing down alcohol absorption.

On the other hand, the carbon dioxide in sparkling wine or some mixed drinks actually speeds up absorption, which is what gives champagne its reputation for making people drunk. Also, the higher the alcohol content of the beverage, the faster your blood alcohol level rises.

TEENS SPEAK

"I Just Had One Glass"

Heather won't soon forget the experiment in alcohol absorption which she "performed" last December. Her older sister, Sid, was taking her and her parents out for dinner but wanted to stop off first at her office's Christmas party.

Heather is 15, but she's a little shy in a room full of strangers, so she stood against the wall near the exit to wait for her parents to show up. Unfortunately, that was right near the punch bowl. "I just had one glass. It was delicious, like pop, and anyway Sid had told me it wasn't very alcoholic—two parts wine to one part fruit juice and one part seltzer water. We were expecting my parents any minute. But then ten minutes passed, and I started getting fidgety.

"I didn't want to eat anything from the buffet and spoil my appetite, so I took another glass of punch. After all, I've had two glasses of wine before, at Thanksgiving dinner, without any problem.

"But those two drinks one after the other, on an empty stomach, with all those bubbles, were a killer. It all went to my head in no time flat; I got so woozy I almost fell flat on my face. Sid and her boss had to walk me to the ladies' room to lie down. I felt so stupid, but I learned my lesson. I'm glad I was with nice people when it happened."

An individual's size matters too. If two individuals have the same type of drink, an individual weighing 200 pounds has a blood alcohol level that is half of someone who weighs 100 pounds. But the heavier guy retains the alcohol in his system longer, since his extra weight slows down the alcohol's elimination.

Men and women also absorb alcohol differently. Men have enzymes (active chemicals) in the stomach, which help break down alcohol before it can be absorbed. These enzymes are much less active in women. In addition, men's bodies tend to have a higher ratio of water to fatty tissue, so that the water in their body tissues dilutes some of the alcohol.

In other words, if a man and a woman of the same body weight have the same type of drink, the woman absorbs more alcohol into her bloodstream (30 percent more, by some estimates), and the alcohol she does absorb does not get diluted as much. Of course, the average woman is smaller than the average man, so the difference in BAC, or blood alcohol levels, is even greater, on the average, between men and women having the same type and amount of alcohol.

Differences in the reproductive systems of men and women also affect alcohol absorption. Women seem to absorb more alcohol into their blood during the premenstrual phase (just before a period). Women who take birth control pills also have higher levels of absorption.

One other important note for women: Alcohol has no trouble finding its way into breast milk. Any mother who is breast-feeding her newborn child should avoid alcohol.

Breakdown

Like everything you eat or drink, alcohol has to be metabolized, or broken down into chemicals the body can handle as nutrients or waste. This process takes place mostly in the liver, which removes as much alcohol from the bloodstream as it can at a time. Under normal circumstances, the liver takes about one hour to metabolize the alcohol in one standard-sized drink, whether beer, wine, or liquor.

If you drink more than one drink per hour, the liver does not absorb much of the excess. The alcohol keeps right on circulating through your brain and other organs, creating numerous effects on various parts of your body.

Heavy drinkers may develop some **tolerance** (the ability to handle larger amounts), as the liver becomes able to metabolize alcohol at a higher rate. But this strains the liver, which in turn can have other harmful effects.

EATING, DRINKING, AND CAFFEINE

Most of what people take into their bodies is classified as food—the fuel for the human machine. Normally, scientists consider alcoholic beverages to be drugs rather than foods.

Harmful Effects of Alcohol on Nutrition

Too much alcohol:

- Causes pancreas to send fewer enzymes to stomach →
  Stomach fails to digest (break down) nutrients

- Damages stomach wall →
  Stomach fails to absorb enough nutrients
  Gastrointestinal bleeding →
    Loss of iron
  Stomach doesn't absorb enough vitamins →
    Thiamine deficiency can damage brain
    Folate vitamin deficiency alters lining of small intestine →
      Small intestine less able to absorb water, sodium, glucose

- Impairs insulin secretion →
  Can cause low blood sugar in undernourished people

- Prevents glucose formation from protein →
  Brain and other tissues starved of glucose

- Impairs digestion, synthesis, and processing of protein →
  Inadequate protein impairs cell structure

- Impairs fat absorption →
  Less absorption of calcium
  Less absorption of vitamins A, E, and D, which are normally
  absorbed along with fat →
    Vitamin A deficiency affects vision, and
    Vitamin D deficiency causes softening of bones

- Liver stores less vitamins

- Liver produces less protein, protein synthesis impaired →
  Cell structure damaged

Source: U.S. Department of Health and Human Services, 2009.

Alcohol and nutrition

Alcohol does contain calories, however, which the body can use, while beer and wine provide traces (very small amounts) of nutrients. So what happens if you compare alcohol to food, for the sake of argument? How does it stack up? Not very well. You may have heard that red wine contains iron, but you'd need to drink about 30 glasses a day to get all the iron you need. And calcium? Fifty 12-ounce cans of beer give you all the calcium your bones could desire in a day.

The one food value that moderate drinking provides is calories—an average of 210 per drink. But today's teenagers get plenty of calories already. Also, alcohol instructs the liver to produce fat at a higher rate. Excess fat (from alcohol or any other source) winds up as deposits of unsightly **adipose tissue,** commonly known as flab. If your diet is already providing you with enough calories, you may put on a pound of fat by having 17 drinks over the course of one month.

On the other hand, heavy drinkers do not necessarily gain weight, even though half the calories they consume may come from alcohol. First of all, more of the energy from alcohol (compared with other calorie sources) gets burned up as heat rather than stored as fat. Moreover, alcohol can cause serious nutritional problems that work against weight gain. Unfortunately, alcoholics often neglect their diet too, making nutritional problems even worse.

Alcohol can slow down the absorption of some vital nutrients, such as vitamins A, B1, B12, C, D, E, and folic acid. As a result, these vitamins are eliminated as waste via the digestive system before the body can use them. Even moderate drinkers should be especially careful to eat a nutritious diet.

Alcohol also can affect the metabolism of protein, leading to the loss of muscle fiber. And if that isn't enough, it also reduces the breakdown of fats. To put it bluntly, heavy drinking often leads to malnutrition, although scientists are still not sure why alcohol has these effects.

Alcohol and coffee

When drinkers want to sober up, they often turn to one of the most widely used drugs in the world—caffeine. In other words, the caffeine in a strong cup of coffee is also a kind of drug, though much milder than alcohol.

Combining alcohol and caffeine may be a mistake. It is true that caffeine, whether in a cup of coffee or in certain over-the-counter painkillers, can stimulate the nervous system, including the brain. Taken in small doses when you are sober, it can make you feel more alert and energetic and can keep you awake.

Caffeine, however, has no power to reduce the level of alcohol in your bloodstream or your brain. Nor does it interact with alcohol in any way to reduce its effects. That cup of coffee may make you feel a bit more sober, but the alcohol is still working in the same way, and your reaction time is still below par. Mixing a **stimulant** (caffeine) and a **depressant** (alcohol) is a recipe for trouble. It may give you a false sense of security and mislead you into thinking you can drive safely.

Besides, too much caffeine can make anyone jittery and restless. When you combine the two drugs in your bloodstream, the results are unpredictable. One thing is sure: If you feel drunk enough to want to sober up, coffee simply does *not* make you capable of driving or reacting safely.

THE EFFECTS OF ALCOHOL AND MEDICATIONS
More than 2,800 prescription drugs are on the market in the United States and another 2,000 over-the-counter medications are available without a prescription. Many of these medicines should never be mixed with alcohol.

If the package label for any medicine—prescription or over-the-counter—says "not to be taken with alcohol," believe it. Alcohol can make that drug either useless or dangerous.

Bad interactions range from the mildly upsetting to the deadly. They generally fall into four types: those that enhance the intoxicating effects of alcohol; those that enhance the intended effects of the medication; those that inhibit or neutralize the intended effects of the medication; and alcohol-medication combinations that are toxic and potentially fatal. Here is a brief look at some of the more common or serious interactions.

Antibiotics are medications used to treat infections. Combined with alcohol, some may cause headaches, nausea, vomiting, and even convulsions. The effectiveness of others is reduced when combined with alcohol.

Antidepressant medications can help reduce antisocial behavior, anxiety, depression, eating disorders, insomnia, obsessive/compulsive disorders, and panic attacks. Doctors prescribe them for many adolescents and teens. This class of drug enhances the intoxicating effects of alcohol. At the same time, alcohol increases the sedating effects of most antidepressants, causing drowsiness, dizziness, and poor coordination.

Beer and red wine are in a special category when it comes to antidepressants. They contain a chemical called tyramine that dangerously interacts with a class of antidepressant drugs called MAOIs (monoamine oxidase inhibitors) to cause a potentially fatal increase in blood pressure.

Alcohol also increases the sedating effects of antihistamines, such as Benadryl, used to treat allergies; antipsychotics, such as Thorazine, used to treat delusions and convulsions; prescription pain relievers, such as codeine and Demerol; sedatives, such as Valium, used to treat anxiety; and hypnotics (sleeping pills), prescribed for sleep disorders.

Combining alcohol with certain heart medications and antiseizure drugs can significantly reduce the benefits of these prescribed medications and put people with heart disease and epilepsy, respectively, at serious risk.

Finally, the combination of alcohol and the most widely taken over-the-counter pain reliever—**acetaminophen** (sold under various brand names, including Tylenol)—can cause serious liver damage and even liver failure.

The bottom line when it comes to alcohol and medication is this: Avoid alcohol and always know what you are taking, why you are taking it, and what its possible side effects may be.

THINGS YOU CAN SEE

If you need to know whether someone has been drinking or has a drinking problem, you won't be able to tell by wondering about his or her metabolism or the activity of the stomach enzymes. But alcohol does have visible effects on the body that can serve to tip off friends or family members who care to be observant.

Effects on behavior

Subtle signs can let you know that people are under the influence of alcohol—even if they are not obviously intoxicated. Other symptoms may indicate a persistent drinking problem.

Many people can have one or two alcoholic drinks without losing their ability to perform routine, simple physical and mental tasks. But with each increased dose of alcohol, more complicated tasks become harder to carry out, even for people who don't act as if they are drunk or intoxicated. For example, any work requiring hand-eye coordination suffers—even something as simple as picking up a pen from the floor.

People under the influence of alcohol often have difficulty doing more than one thing at a time. They may talk clearly or walk without swaying, but they focus what attention they have on only one task at a time. They can be easily distracted and may have trouble remembering things. Their reaction times may suffer—which is what makes it so risky to drive "under the influence." And they may talk or behave in a manner that is inappropriate to the situation—for example, laughing, crying, or arguing over trivial details.

Of course, even when sober, some people are highly focused while others are more relaxed and easygoing. Some people have a steel-trap memory for detail, while others cheerfully admit, with a smile and a shrug, that they just cannot remember names. But it is the change from normal behavior that can be a sign of intoxication.

A drinker's eyes can be a giveaway too. Sometimes the signs are obvious. Alcohol can cause congestion of the blood vessels (too much blood) in the eye, so that the whites appear bloodshot and irritated. Or the eyes may appear overly moist and "glassy," or even unmoving and lifeless.

Some of the signs are less obvious, and may be difficult to catch at first glance. For example: When you are sober, your brain has an astonishing ability to focus and refocus your eye muscles as you move your head or as different objects come into view. Alcohol can slow down this complex mental function. A person who has had too much to drink often experiences blurred or double vision. When people struggle to see something within their normal range, too much alcohol may be the reason.

Even moderate drinking can have an affect on the eyes. For example, usually someone who looks to the side while holding his or her head still has no difficulty doing so. When someone who has been drinking tries it, the eyeballs often twitch or vibrate noticeably. Experiments have shown that the higher the level of blood alcohol, the less the eye has to move sideways in order to trigger this effect. Moderate drinkers may learn to compensate for these effects, for example, by turning their bodies toward you when you speak, rather than just their eyes.

Q & A

Question: Is it true that alcohol can shrink the brain?

Answer: Unfortunately, yes. Autopsies have long shown that people with chronic alcohol problems have smaller and lighter brains. CAT scans and MRIs of live patients show the same effects. When alcoholics who continue to drink are monitored over several years, their brains appear to get progressively smaller. The effect seems to be most severe in the outer layer of the frontal lobe, which controls higher intelligence.

Effects on the skin

Alcohol consumption can make some people's skin turn red. When the liver breaks down alcohol, one of the chemicals it produces along the way is **acetaldehyde.** This fairly toxic chemical is eventually broken down into acetic acid, which is harmless and can even be used to store energy. But as long as acetaldehyde is circulating through the bloodstream, it works its effects—increased heart rate, impaired judgment, and a redness or flushing in the face (caused by an increased flow, or "flush," of blood).

Some people have a reduced capacity to break down acetaldehyde. Even one drink turns their face visibly red; it also makes them feel ill. This trait is especially common in Chinese, Japanese, and Koreans, and among Asian Americans. But it happens to people of other backgrounds as well. Few such people ever become alcoholic—if a couple of drinks make you feel ill, you probably do not want to keep drinking.

Alcohol has still another unsightly affect on the skin—frequent bruises. They are not just the result of bumping into tables or door frames. Alcohol has a harmful effect on the body's ability to handle internal bleeding after an injury. Normally, sticky blood cells, called **platelets,** rush to the site of a wound and form miniscule clots, which keep the blood from leaking out of the artery into the surrounding tissue. Lab tests show that heavy drinkers have lower than normal levels of platelets. If the wound is near the surface of the body, blood seeps out under the skin, causing a visible red or black bruise.

A few people are even allergic to alcohol, or to some of the other ingredients in beer or wine. They may develop hives from only one drink.

More common than allergies is rosacea, a condition where the face becomes permanently red and pimply, especially on or around the nose. Alcohol is only one of many causes of this condition; but severe cases, where the nose becomes enlarged and bulbous (or bumpy), are often caused or aggravated by long-term heavy drinking.

Fact Or Fiction?

Alcohol warms up the body on a cold day.

The Facts: The truth is just the opposite. After a few drinks, the blood vessels near the skin expand, giving you a flushed sensation, which feels warm against the cold. However, this means that your body is losing heat through the skin, heat that you really need internally. This is how drunk people can freeze to death from exposure.

SO MANY EFFECTS

Alcohol is a powerful drug that can dramatically affect a person's mood and behavior. No one should be surprised that it also produces a long list of physical changes to the drinker's body. Anyone who decides to drink should keep these effects in mind, and act sensibly to keep the risk of harm to a minimum.

See also: Alcohol Abuse, The Risks of; Alcohol and Disease; Tolerance and Reverse Tolerance

FURTHER READING

Bellenir, Karen, ed. *Substance Abuse Sourcebook.* Detroit, Mich.: Omnigraphics, 1996.

Haring, Raymond V. *Myths, Mysteries and Management of Alcohol.* Sacramento, Calif.: HealthSpan, 1995.

Miller, William R., and Kathleen M. Carroll. *Rethinking Substance Abuse: What the Science Shows, and What We Should Do About It.* New York: The Guilford Press, 2006.

Wolff, Lisa. *Issues in Alcohol.* San Diego, Calif.: Lucent, 1999.

■ ENABLING BEHAVIORS

See: Codependency

■ ETHNICITY AND ALCOHOL

Racial and group differences in the use of alcohol and the problems associated with drinking. Alcohol use, alcohol-related problems,

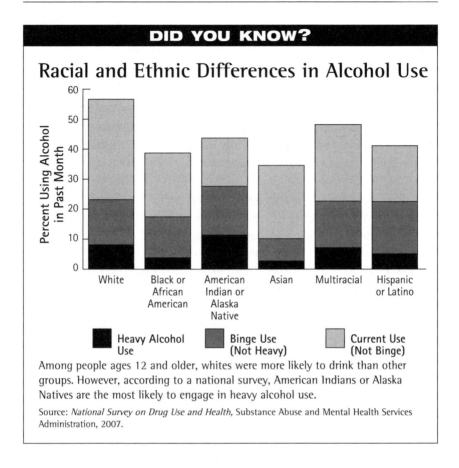

DID YOU KNOW?

Racial and Ethnic Differences in Alcohol Use

Among people ages 12 and older, whites were more likely to drink than other groups. However, according to a national survey, American Indians or Alaska Natives are the most likely to engage in heavy alcohol use.

Source: *National Survey on Drug Use and Health,* Substance Abuse and Mental Health Services Administration, 2007.

and treatment for alcohol abuse vary by race and population group. Generally speaking, whites are more likely to both use and abuse alcohol than any other group. They are also more likely to have access to alcohol-treatment programs.

ALCOHOL USE BY DIFFERENT GROUPS

According to the 2008 edition of the study "Monitoring the Future," among 12th-grade students, whites are more likely to drink than blacks or Hispanics. Almost 30 percent of white 12th-grade students reported having five or more drinks in the previous two weeks. This compares to 11.5 percent of black students and 22.5 percent of Hispanic students. Also, when examining trends in a 30-day period of drinking beer, 41 percent of white students admitted to using alcohol. Only 13.6 percent of black students and 32.7 percent of Hispanic students said they had drunk a beer. White students were also more likely to get drunk—33.7 percent had been drunk in the past 30 days. Twenty-four percent of Hispanic students and 14.6 percent of black students indicated they had been drunk.

PREDICTORS OF ALCOHOL ABUSE

The authors of a 2007 study in the *American Journal on Addictions* examined racial and ethnic differences in what predicts alcohol abuse in adolescents. The researchers studied adolescents who were admitted to a hospital for psychiatric treatment. This allowed the authors to see what psychological factors influenced alcohol abuse and then how the adolescents differed by race. For whites, who were classified as European Americans, the following helped predict alcohol abuse: self-esteem, age, impulsiveness, peer insecurity, childhood abuse, and predispositions toward delinquent behavior. For Latinos, there were only two factors that helped predict alcohol abuse: predisposition toward delinquency and childhood abuse. For African Americans, none of the factors the authors looked at predicted alcohol abuse. These results make it clear that the same factors do not influence behavior in the same way across races.

A 2003 report by the National Institute on Alcohol Abuse and Alcoholism (NIAAA) presented factors that increase or decrease the risk of using and abusing alcohol among ethnic minorities. For black men, the authors found there were no factors that increased the risk of frequent heavy drinking. However, there were several factors that helped decrease this risk. For example, both retirement and religion were important. Black men who were retired or stated that religion was important in their lives were less likely to be heavy and frequent drinkers. However, the authors found that black women were exposed to risk factors. Being unemployed or having a lower income increased the odds of frequent heavy drinking. Age was seen as a protective factor; older women (over age 50) were less likely to drink than younger black women (18–29).

For Hispanics, unemployment was a risk factor for both men and women. Hispanic women who were unemployed were at an increased risk for drinking when compared to those women who were employed. Similarly with black men, Hispanic women were at less of a risk for frequent heavy drinking if they were retired and indicated that religion played an important role in their lives.

Racial and ethnic differences in alcohol use and related problems can be explained by several factors. Norms and attitudes play an important role. For example, the authors of the 2003 NIAA report indicate that Hispanics and blacks hold more conservative attitudes regarding alcohol use.

One group that has received only minimal attention when it comes to drinking problems is Asians. The authors of a 2008 study in the *Journal of Studies on Alcohol and Drugs* examined the differences in alcohol use between Korean and Chinese college students. They found that Korean students drank more often and more heavily than Chinese students. For example, Korean students averaged six drinks a week, while Chinese students averaged only three drinks a week. When looking at the maximum number of drinks consumed on any one occasion, Korean students also drank more than Chinese students—six drinks to three drinks. This means that when looking at the most a student drank on any one occasion, Korean students drank twice as much as Chinese students.

In another study, the authors of a 2004 article in *Ethnicity and Health* examined ethnic differences in alcohol use among students in London, England. The researchers looked at differences between blacks of Caribbean descent, blacks of African descent, English whites, and Irish whites. The authors also included gender differences. (It is important to know that in England, women are slightly more likely to drink than men.) In this study, 88.6 percent of English white males had at least one drink in their lives, compared to 88.1 percent of Irish white males, 79.6 percent of Caribbean blacks, and 50 percent of African blacks. The same overall pattern holds for women—94.6 percent of Irish white females drank, followed by English white females (89.1 percent), Caribbean black females (81.4 percent), and African black females (49.1 percent). White males and females were more likely to have been drunk at least once in the past 90 days, as well as at least once a week in the past 90 days.

ALCOHOL-RELATED PROBLEMS

Alcohol use and abuse can lead to social, economic, legal, and physical problems. Just as there are racial and ethnic differences in alcohol use, there are also differences in exposure to the problems that stem from alcohol use and abuse. Problems include relationship conflicts, difficulty with schoolwork, job issues, trouble with the law, physical problems, and many more.

Marital status is also a factor in experiencing alcohol-related problems. In a 2003 NIAAA report, the authors found that whites are less likely to have such problems if they are married, when compared to those who are divorced, separated, or never married. Black men, on the other hand, are more likely to experience alcohol-related problems if they are married when compared to those who are widowed. Hispanic men who are unemployed or earn a low income (less than $10,000 per year) are at an increased risk of experiencing alcohol-related problems.

A child's exposure to alcohol-related problems also varies according to race. In a 2004 study in the *Journal of Studies on Alcohol,* the authors found that the proportion of white children exposed to alcohol-related problems was lower than the proportion of black or Hispanic children who are exposed to drinking problems. Only 14.5 percent of white children were exposed to these problems, whereas approximately 19 percent of both Hispanic and black children were exposed to alcohol-related problems.

DRIVING WHILE INTOXICATED

Driving under the influence of alcohol (DUI) is one of the very serious problems that stems from drinking. The authors of a 2005 study in the journal *Accident Analysis and Prevention* found racial and ethnic differences for reports of DUI. Twenty-two percent of white men admitted to driving under the influence, compared to 16.5 percent of blacks and 16.8 percent of Hispanics. White women also were more likely to drive under the influence when compared to black and Hispanic women. Whereas 11.8 percent of white women admitted to DUI, 9.2 and 6.7 percent of black and Hispanic women, respectively, admitted to DUI. Being arrested for DUI, however, occurred most frequently for Hispanic men, followed next by black men and then by white men. Regardless of race, women were rarely arrested for DUI. Among women, black women were most likely to be arrested for DUI. However, it should be noted that only 0.4 percent of black women were arrested for DUI. The group of women that is most likely to be arrested only gets arrested less than one-half of 1 percent of the time.

In an earlier study in the journal *Accident Analysis and Prevention* in 2000, researchers had also examined racial differences in DUI. The results were similar—white men (22 percent) were more likely to drive under the influence than Hispanic (21 percent) or black men (11 percent). Four percent of Hispanic men were arrested for DUI compared to 1 percent for both white and black men.

FETAL ALCOHOL SYNDROME

FAS is a serious alcohol-related problem for infants whose mothers drink during pregnancy. Symptoms of FAS include low birth weight, failure to thrive, behavioral problems, developmental delays, and organs failing to work properly. A 2008 study in *Maternal and Child Health Journal* presented data on the reduction of drinking during pregnancy. The authors found that, overall, white women were significantly more likely to reduce their alcohol consumption during their pregnancy. Black, Hispanic, and Asian women were less likely to do so.

TREATMENT FOR ALCOHOL ABUSE

The authors of a 2007 study in the journal *Alcoholism: Clinical and Experimental Research* examined national data to see what racial differences exist in using services available to treat people with drinking problems. The authors found that 5.4 percent of whites had sought help for alcohol problems. Only 4.5 percent of both blacks and Hispanics indicated that they had sought help. When focusing on people with alcohol abuse or dependence, 16.3 percent of blacks indicated they sought help. This figure is lower for both whites and Hispanics—15.8 percent and 14.7 percent of these groups, respectively, had sought help.

Approximately the same percentage of whites and blacks sought help from a specialty program—9.6 and 9.0 percent, respectively. Only 5.7 percent of Hispanics sought help from specialty programs. Alcoholics Anonymous was equally popular among all three groups.

Q & A

Question: Do members of different races and ethnicities have the same access to alcohol treatment programs?

Answer: Barriers to treatment for some groups do exist. Part of the reason for racial differences in receiving help involves access to resources. The 2007 study in *Alcoholism: Clinical and Experimental Research* indicated that these barriers were more of a problem for Hispanics than for whites. Finding services and paying for services and child care were cited as reasons that made it difficult or impossible to get help by 58 percent of Hispanics who wanted treatment.

The authors of a 2008 study in the *Journal of Clinical Psychiatry* examined racial differences in treatment for those who had substance-abuse problems, including alcohol, and mood or anxiety disorders. Although whites were significantly more likely than blacks to receive help for mood disorders (52.7 percent versus 35.2 percent), there were no racial differences in seeking treatment for alcohol disorders. There was no more than a 1.1 percent difference between whites and blacks when it came to seeking different types of treatment for alcoholism. Treatment types included 12-step programs, using alcohol-specific programs, social-service programs, and going to a hospital's emergency department for help.

See also: Birth Defects and Alcohol; Screening for Alcoholism

FURTHER READING
Lala, Shulamith, and Ashenberg Straussner. *Ethnocultural Factors in Substance Abuse Treatment.* New York: The Guilford Press, 2002.

■ HANGOVER

A catchall term referring to the nasty physical symptoms people typically have the day after drinking a large quantity of alcohol. Once you have one, you will never forget how it feels. With any luck—and a little good sense—you will never suffer the health problems of an alcoholic. But unless you abstain from alcohol all your life, sooner or later you probably will have a hangover.

You don't need to be a heavy drinker to suffer from hangovers. In fact, light and moderate drinkers are the most likely to suffer, according to a report appearing in 2000 in the *Annals of Internal Medicine.* Inexperienced and first-time drinkers are also at risk, until they learn their "limit."

Hangovers are not only unpleasant to the drinker on the morning after. They can have serious effects on other people too. They cause more economic damage in the workplace—through absenteeism, lost wages, or poor job performance—than any other alcohol-related factor. Hangovers also are an important cause of neglect and child abuse by alcoholic parents: The hours spent laying in bed in misery cannot be devoted to caring for a child's physical and emotional needs.

SIGNS, SYMPTOMS, AND CAUSES

The most common symptoms of hangover are mild to severe headache, nausea or stomach pain and vomiting, a dry mouth and thirst, muscle aches, physical and mental fatigue, dizziness, sensitivity to noise, light, and movement, sweating, tremors, and unpleasant emotions such as irritability, anxiety, and even depression.

If you experience all of these together, you may resolve then and there never to abuse alcohol again. More often, however, people experience only some of the symptoms, depending on the individual's personal body chemistry, the type and quantity of alcoholic beverage he or she drank, and perhaps the person's state of mind when drinking. As a general rule of thumb, though, the more alcohol you drink, the more likely you are to have a hangover.

A lot of different things go on in your body to cause so many different symptoms. One researcher sums it up as "dehydration; metabolic acidosis; hypoglycemia; disturbed prostaglandin synthesis; abnormal secretion of vasopressin, cortisol, aldosterone, renin, and testosterone; increased cardiac output; tachycardia; and vasodilatation." Translated into plain English, he means: The body has too little water, too much acid, not enough blood sugar, too much or too little of various powerful hormones, too much blood pumped out of the heart at too fast a rate, and dilation (widening) of the arteries. Quite a lot for just a few drinks!

Hangovers are considered a kind of alcohol **withdrawal,** the **syndrome** (set of symptoms) that alcoholics experience when they try to stop drinking or when they are unable to obtain another drink.

By the time the symptoms of a hangover are at their peak, very little **ethanol** (the chemical name for alcohol) or its direct breakdown product, **acetaldehyde,** is left in the body. But the alcohol has already done its "work" by causing dehydration, or the reduction in the body's water supply. Ethanol is a diuretic, a substance that gets the kidneys to drain water away from other organs. That draining causes the dryness and thirst, and probably contributes to the headache as well.

If alcohol itself is no longer in the body, what creates the other symptoms? **Congeners,** or impurities, are probably responsible for many of them. These organic chemicals are produced as a by-product of the manufacture of beer, wine, and distilled spirits (liquors). They stay in the barrel or bottle, helping to give each beverage its distinctive flavor. Some of the chief congeners are **histamines**, types of congeners found in alcoholic beverages that cause reactions in people who are allergic, and **methanol**, a congener that adds flavor to alcoholic beverages; another, found in red wine, is **tyramine**, a congener that can be dangerous for a drinker who also takes antidepressants and can cause headaches all by itself.

Some researchers now say that methanol is the chief culprit. Methanol is found in higher quantities in the types of beverages that usually cause the worst hangovers, such as champagne and inexpensive whiskeys. Furthermore, the time it takes the body to break down methanol into its toxic components—formaldehyde and formic acid—is about the same amount of time it takes for a hangover to kick in after you finish drinking. Finally, people whose bodies break down methanol faster seem to suffer the most.

Your hangover may be worse if you are tired or "overdo it" while you are drinking. As you drink, you become less sensitive to your own body. You probably don't pay attention to your body's signals that you need to stop partying and go to sleep. Even without alcohol, physical exhaustion can cause some of the same symptoms as a hangover.

Your general state of health and nutrition matters too. A healthy body is better equipped to handle a temporary "assault" such as too much alcohol.

Finally, your state of mind may have an effect. A study reported in the *Journal of Clinical Epidemiology* in 1993 confirmed the traditional belief that those who drink alcohol when they are angry, anxious, or depressed are more likely to suffer from hangovers.

Fact Or Fiction?

As long as you don't "mix drinks," you won't get a hangover.

The Facts: There is no evidence that mixing different kinds or brands of alcoholic beverages has any effect on hangovers. You can get a nightmarish hangover even if you stick with one drink all night—provided you drink enough of it and the other factors are present. And if people only have a few drinks, properly diluted and spaced over a pleasant evening of food and sociability, they may well avoid any hangover even if, for example, they combined a predinner vodka cocktail, a small glass of draft beer at the table, and a splash of dessert wine in the living room.

PREVENTION

To state the obvious, the best way to avoid a hangover is not to drink, or not to have more than one or two drinks at any one time. However, drinkers can take some other steps to reduce the likelihood and the severity of a hangover.

First of all, avoid drinks with high amounts of congeners. Champagne and inexpensive whiskeys have the highest, followed by tequila, brandy, bourbon, and red wine. Clear rum, better whiskeys, and white wine usually cause fewer or less severe hangovers, and gin, vodka, and beer (especially pale beers and light beers) cause even fewer. Gin and vodka are popular with many alcoholics, possibly for this reason.

Many theories have been advanced to try to explain these variations between beverages. Some of the theories even contradict one another. Here are a few: The longer a beverage ages, the more congeners form and the more likely the drinker will get a hangover; expensive liquors that are distilled several times are likely to be freer of the impurities that cause hangovers; prestigious "single malt" scotches cause worse hangovers than cheaper "blends."

The more experts you turn to, the more complicated the list becomes, perhaps too complicated. For most people, learning to drink responsibly—or not at all—will prevent more hangovers than all the research into congeners in the world.

People who drink hard liquor, such as whiskey, gin, bourbon, or vodka, should always dilute it with ice and a noncarbonated liquid such as water or juice (carbonation makes the stomach absorb alcohol faster). In addition, "topping off" a drink now and then with more mixer helps lessen the amount of alcohol one drinks overall. When it is diluted in the stomach, each dose of alcohol takes more time to enter the bloodstream. The mixers also help restore some of the water that alcohol drains from the body.

Drinking water is another popular preventive measure that seems to work for most people. Some advise drinkers to down a couple of glasses of water before going to sleep. Others say to drink one glass of water—larger than the wine or liquor glass—after each drink. Drinking water replaces some of the fluids drained away by alcohol, thus avoiding those symptoms caused by dehydration, possibly even headaches.

If a bad frame of mind contributes to hangovers, a person is better off drinking with friends or family in a pleasant environment rather than drinking alone at home or in a bar surrounded by cigarette smoke. That might be safer and healthier for other reasons (for one thing, your friends might keep you from driving); avoiding hangovers would just be an added bonus.

Experts do not agree on the value of painkillers or food supplements, such as vitamins, in preventing hangovers. Some experts warn against aspirin, the most popular choice, because it can irritate the stomach lining, which may already be inflamed by alcohol. Fizzy aspirin, such as Alka Seltzer, may offer a better alternative, since it spends less time in the stomach.

Acetaminophen (the medicine in Tylenol and similar products) may actually harm the liver if taken after having several alcoholic drinks. Acetaminophen by itself can be dangerous in large doses (higher than the number recommended on the label). When the liver is weakened by alcohol, even a few tablets can be toxic.

Some people swear by vitamins, amino acids, or herbs; others make money by packaging these common supplements in special "hangover prevention" form. Remember, unlike pharmaceutical (drug) companies, the makers of these products do not need to get government approval for their health claims. It is probably foolhardy to think that taking these products will allow you to ignore the practical steps of hangover prevention already discussed.

TREATMENT

A fully effective treatment for alcohol hangovers may never be found, according to one 1997 report in the *British Medical Journal*. The reason? The syndrome has too many different causes, and it affects too many different parts of the body.

Some doctors also fear that an effective next-day treatment would do more harm than good by masking the unhealthy effects of overdrinking. They believe unpleasant hangovers may help some drinkers understand the damage they are inflicting on their bodies. Such people may then learn to control or eliminate their bad drinking habits and avoid more serious, long-term damage.

However, some partial treatments may help. It often helps to drink lots of water the morning after, to restore your body's water balance. Sufferers can also try over-the-counter pain relievers other than acetaminophen (see the warnings in the "Prevention" section above).

When studied by scientists, some traditional remedies do not seem to work at all. Cups of steaming hot coffee, cold showers, or exercise do little or no good. But sugary tea, a time-honored folk remedy, may help counteract the effects of low blood sugar.

The most dangerous "cure" is perhaps the most famous one—"the hair of the dog that bit you." This cliché means that a person who wakes up with a horrible hangover should have a fresh alcoholic drink to deaden the pain.

There is a scientific explanation why this temporary "cure" might work. The alcohol in the "new" drink keeps the liver from breaking down the methanol from the old drink into the toxic chemicals that may cause hangover symptoms. Unfortunately, the new drink has its own supply of methanol and other congeners, and the whole unpleasant cycle begins again.

Bottom line: When you have a hangover, your body has just gone through the mill. All systems need to rest, at least for several hours. For severe hangovers, researchers recommend a good 72-hour break before taking a single drink.

In fact, starting the day with an "eye-opener," or morning drink, is one of the sure signs of a developing alcohol dependency. More than a few alcoholics finally understood that they had a problem when they felt themselves reaching for a bottle as soon as they woke up.

If the sensible treatments don't seem to help, get back into bed, if at all possible, and sleep it off. Time may not heal all wounds, as the saying goes, but it definitely does "cure" a hangover.

TAKE IT AS A WARNING

A hangover is neither funny nor trivial. The pain, misery, and disruption it brings can serve as a hint of the long-term dangers of alcohol. Smart people take the hint and learn to behave sensibly in the future.

See also: Alcohol Abuse, The Risks of, Alcohol and Depression

FURTHER READING

Haring, Raymond V. *Myths, Mysteries, and Management of Alcohol.* Sacramento, Calif.: HealthSpan Communications, 1995.
Stewart, Gail. *Teen Alcoholics.* San Diego, Calif.: Lucent Books, 2000.

■ LAW AND DRINKING, THE

Alcohol laws have been around almost as long as alcohol itself. Even ancient civilizations regulated the sale and public consumption of alcohol, and so have most governments since. At the same time, the beverage has been an important source of government revenue through taxes or monopolies.

The United States is no exception to this rule. The first colonists who arrived from England brought with them a set of beliefs about alcohol and how to control its use. These beliefs have gone through many changes, and have generated years of passionate controversy. In response, the laws have been repeatedly changed, at the federal, state, and local levels. And because the American population and public opinion are constantly changing, alcohol laws are likely to change again.

TEMPERANCE MOVEMENT

Though many of the English colonists who came to America were strict observers of religious law, they were not abstainers, or nondrinkers. The famous Puritan preacher Increase Mather wrote, "Drink is in itself a good creature of God, but the abuse of drink is from Satan." The colonists produced and consumed large quantities of beer, whiskey, gin, and rum. In fact, rum was probably the most valuable product manufactured in the colonies. Local governments encouraged the licensing and building of breweries, distilleries, and taverns.

After the United States became independent, the first major threat to its unity was the so-called Whiskey Rebellion of 1794. Thousands of farmers in western Pennsylvania refused to honor a new federal tax on liquor, which they felt threatened their freedom to produce and consume as much whiskey as they chose.

By the early 1800s, Americans were drinking about three times as much liquor, beer, and wine as they do today, and alcohol abuse was commonplace. In reaction, a **temperance movement** began to emerge, especially among churchgoers. The movement condemned alcohol abuse as a source of disease and poverty. As alternatives, it promoted temperance, or moderation, in drinking, and encouraged the use of nonalcoholic beverages such as root beer.

It was an era of reformist movements, such as abolitionism (which opposed slavery), prison reform, and women's rights. Many women were active in the temperance movement, which spread throughout United States and to many European countries.

By the middle of the 1800s, the movement began to advocate **prohibition**—a complete ban on the sale or drinking of alcohol. Maine became the first state to outlaw alcohol, in 1851, and several other states followed.

The founding of the Prohibition Party in 1869 and the Women's Christian Temperance Union in 1874 signaled the start of a major political campaign. For the next 60 years, alcohol remained one of the most important issues on the political agenda, affecting every presidential election for decades. The issues split the country into regional, religious, and urban or rural factions.

In the early 1900s, the movement gained support from social reformers who wanted to protect the working classes from alcoholism, political reformers who saw alcohol and taverns as a key part of corrupt political machines, and business owners looking to reduce absenteeism and injuries in their factories.

VOLSTEAD ACT OF 1919

During World War I (1917–18), the government declared wartime prohibition, in part to divert grain from alcohol production to food. Then, in 1919, the Eighteenth Amendment to the U.S. Constitution was ratified, outlawing the "manufacture, sale and transportation of intoxicating liquors." Later that year Congress passed the famous **Volstead Act,** which put the amendment into effect. What people called "the great experiment" of Prohibition was under way.

The Volstead Act defined "intoxicating liquors" as any beverage whose alcohol content was 0.5 percent or more, which made beer and wine, as well as hard liquor, illegal. But the Eighteenth Amendment did not make it illegal to possess liquor for personal use, and the Volstead Act did not generally allow searches of individual homes. As a result, many people began to make their own alcoholic beverages. Businesses could legally produce alcohol for industrial and scientific purposes and for sacramental use, for example by Catholic priests or Jewish rabbis. Doctors also could prescribe wine or liquor for "medicinal" reasons. All these loopholes eventually allowed large quantities of legally manufactured alcohol to be sidetracked for sale by **bootleggers,** the importers and bulk sellers of illegal alcohol, and speak-easies, or illegal saloons.

The federal government set up a Prohibition Bureau in the Treasury Department to enforce the Volstead Act. Some 170,000 saloons were shut down across the country. Contrary to popular belief, Prohibition was successfully enforced in much of the country, and it achieved many of its aims. Arrests for public drunkenness declined dramatically. Hospital admissions for alcoholism, **alcohol psychosis** (an episode of severe mental illness), and alcohol-related diseases fell by more than half within a few years.

Prohibitionists claimed that there were fewer broken homes caused by lost wages and domestic violence. The evidence shows that alcohol consumption fell the most among poorer people, who could not afford the high price of illegal alcohol. Even after Prohibition was repealed by the Twenty-first Amendment, and sales resumed in 1934, consumption did not immediately rise to pre-1919 levels, which suggests that many people had lost the habit of drinking.

The tales of Prohibition crime made popular in many gangster movies have been somewhat exaggerated, according to some historians. Organized criminal mobs ran illegal rackets in the big cities long before Prohibition, and murder rates had already risen well before 1919.

But the law did make millions of ordinary citizens partners in crime. Many immigrant ethnic groups refused to give up their cultural attachment to wine, beer, or whiskey. These drinks also remained an essential part of social life for middle-class people in the cities. Without regulation by the government, much of the alcohol sold was of poor quality, and some was even dangerously toxic.

Fact Or Fiction?

During the 1920s, when Prohibition was in effect in the United States, people drank more than they ever had before.

The Facts: Actually, this is not true. Evidence suggests that there was a sizable reduction in drinking during Prohibition. In many states, alcoholic beverages were not easy to obtain. In all regions, prices went up, and poorer people simply could not afford to drink.

These factors, plus the publicity over Prohibition-related crime and violence, began to make the policy unpopular. When the Great Depression began in 1929, closing factories and throwing millions of people out of work, Prohibition became an economic issue. Opponents held out the hope that repeal would mean new jobs and tax revenues. In

1933, the Twenty-first Amendment to the Constitution was approved, repealing the Eighteenth (Prohibition) Amendment.

Some states continued Prohibition on a statewide or local level; Mississippi was the last state to repeal, in 1966. Most states adopted new laws to limit the sale of alcohol. They restricted the hours and days that taverns could operate, or required taverns to serve food. Some states even banned any sales outside of state-owned "package stores," which never sold by the drink. Many of these laws remain in effect today.

PUBLIC INTOXICATION: CRIMINAL OR VICTIM?

After the repeal of Prohibition, state and local governments continued to deal with alcohol abuse, but their focus shifted. Public intoxication and its dangerous effects once again became the main alcohol-related issue in law and government.

Public drunkenness laws go back more than 300 years, to the first public intoxication statute in England in 1606. In one form or another, these laws always remained on the books, in the United States as well. By the early 1960s, police officers in every state were arresting a total of 2 million people a year for the crime of public intoxication.

However, public opinion had begun to change, partly due to the effort of such groups as **A.A.**, or **Alcoholics Anonymous.** Most people now came to believe that alcoholism should be treated as a disease. They wanted intoxicated people, especially homeless derelicts, to be treated with compassion. They wanted to offer them treatment rather than simply arresting them and allowing them to "dry out" (become sober) in a jail cell.

Despite this public change, the U.S. Supreme Court in 1968 narrowly supported arrests for drunkenness. Partly in response, Congress passed the Alcoholic Rehabilitation Act of 1968. This law was followed two years later by a more comprehensive law that called for major new efforts in research and treatment, and set up the National Institute on Alcohol Abuse and Alcoholism (NIAAA).

Still another 1970s federal law, the Uniform Alcoholism and Intoxication Act, encouraged states to change their approach as well. The majority of states eventually fell in line, removing simple intoxication from the list of crimes, and setting up **detoxification** and rehabilitation programs.

In practice, many public drunks refuse voluntary treatment, and police officers frequently arrest them on "public nuisance" charges. In any case, alcohol researchers have not yet found new, more effective treatment methods for putting a complete stop to alcohol abuse.

In the 1980s, private citizens whose families had suffered from fetal alcohol syndrome and other drinking-related diseases began suing manufacturers and sellers. In response, Congress passed a law requiring health warnings on all alcohol containers.

In July 1984, Congress passed a law setting the national drinking age at 21, and by 1988 all states had adopted the new age requirement. Dramatic and effective campaigns by groups such as Mothers Against Drunk Driving (MADD) helped convince states to raise the minimum drinking age to 21. At the same time, local and state police have worked with judges and juries to strictly enforce drunken driving laws. Following these changes, the rate of fatal alcohol-related car crashes sharply declined.

ZERO TOLERANCE

During the 1980s, the federal government launched a "war on drugs," designed to eliminate the distribution and sale of illegal drugs. It was a response to the alarming increase in drug abuse and addiction, especially among young people.

In that climate, "zero tolerance" became a popular slogan among the public: People wanted the government, school systems, and employers to crack down on *any* violation of the drug laws. For example, they wanted students to be punished, even suspended from school, if they were found with any amount of drugs on school property. Employers began introducing drug tests for new or current employees. Any trace of drugs in urine would be grounds for dismissal.

Over time, the idea spread to other areas of concern, including alcohol. Many states now have zero tolerance for under-21 drivers— they can be prosecuted for having even the smallest non-zero BAL, or blood alcohol level, while driving. Under pressure from parents concerned about a safe, healthy environment for their children, many school systems have issued zero-tolerance policies against alcohol, illegal drugs, violence, and guns.

Q & A

Question: What is the legal drinking age in Canada?

Answer: Each province in Canada regulates alcohol as it sees fit. Three provinces allow drinking at 18: Quebec, Manitoba, and Alberta. All the rest have a legal age of 19. Up until 1970, most provinces maintained a legal minimum of 20 or 21; nine of the 10 provinces lowered the minimum in the early 1970s.

However, some parents, supported by political activists, criticize zero tolerance. They want the government to concentrate on prosecuting the major sellers of illegal drugs rather than the individual users, and they want the schools to focus on alcohol abuses, such as drunkenness or sales on school property.

These opponents have publicized cases of over-eager enforcement, such as the student who was suspended for using mouthwash in the locker room because it contained alcohol (as most popular brands do). Such cases, they say, are evidence of a "prohibition" mentality.

The schools are caught in the middle. Zero-tolerance policies can sometimes be unfair, but they also protect schools against liability (legal responsibility). For example, if a school is sued when a student who drinks on school property is injured, the administration must show that it made every effort to prevent such events from taking place. The controversy continues to spark heated debate.

A BALANCING ACT

Over the centuries, the American legal system has had to adjust to changing currents of public opinion about alcohol. From broad acceptance to prohibition, from a policy of arrest to one of treatment, and now to zero tolerance for young drinkers, the laws have been continually refined. While people still debate the means, most citizens today agree on the goal: to balance the desires of individual to drink against the general interest in health, safety, and public order.

See also: Alcohol and Disease; Drinking and Driving; Ethnicity and Alcohol; Self-Help Programs

FURTHER READING

Barr, Andrew. *Drink: A Social History of America.* New York: Carroll and Graf, 1999.

Flowers, R. Barri. *Drugs, Alcohol and Criminality in American Society.* Jefferson, N.C.: McFarland, 1999.

Kilcommins, Shane. *Alcohol, Society and Law.* West Sussex, U.K.: Barry Rose Law Publishers, 2003.

■ LEGAL ISSUES

See: Law and Drinking, The

■ MEDIA, THE AND ALCOHOL

See: Advertising and Counteradvertising Campaigns

■ PEER PRESSURE AND ALCOHOL

The experience a person has of feeling forced, or compelled, to act the same as the social group to which he or she belongs is known as peer pressure. Face it–everyone likes to belong. Human beings are "social animals," according to scientists. People huddle together for comfort, safety, and because they enjoy one another's company. No one wants to feel left out or excluded from family, class, team, or coworkers.

As social animals, teenagers may be the most "human" of all age groups. They love to hang out with friends, to share good times, to help one another over the rough spots, and to compare notes about all the new things they are finding out about life. There aren't many skills that a teen can learn that are more important than finding and keeping good friends. They deserve your loyalty, and they owe you loyalty in return.

However, people aren't *just* social animals. They are individuals too. An important skill that people need to learn as teens is finding the right balance between belonging to a group and making one's own decisions as an individual. A teen needs to be his or her own person within the family, and among friends too.

LISTENING TO OTHERS

When you were a kid, you probably thought your parents knew everything there was to know. Then, after you spent a few years in school, you realized that they didn't always have all the answers, however much they loved you and however much you respected them. The world had changed a little since they were your age; in some areas, your teachers were the experts now.

Now that you have reached your teens, your life is more complicated. Your parents still have their opinions. Your teachers have their own points of view—and you usually have a new set of teachers every year. You watch television, listen to the radio, and see movies, and you read books, newspapers, and magazines. In addition to all these other sources of information, you have your friends, who are part of your peer group, people your own age in your community.

Your peers are the unchallenged experts in lots of subjects. They usually can tell you the best music to listen to. They know what clothing looks good on you and what looks hopelessly nerdy. They may have a good idea about who the best teachers are in your school, or what part-time jobs are available in your neighborhood. They can even help you navigate through dating, romance, and sex, and keep you from making embarrassing mistakes.

Very often, though, your peers will influence you by their words or by their example, even on subjects where they may not have so much knowledge—for example, alcohol or illegal drugs. There's no reason to *ignore* their opinions, whether on the risks of alcohol or its possible benefits. But they probably do not have the whole picture.

Some of your friends may in fact know some pieces of the puzzle better than your parents or teachers. They may be more familiar with the names and types of the latest "designer" or "club drugs," and where to get them. Your peers may know where underage kids can get alcoholic beverages, and where they can drink with less chance of getting caught. If your parents don't drink much, or don't drink at all, you may have friends that are more knowledgeable about the different types and brands of alcoholic beverages.

Just as your parents "don't know everything," however, your friends can be wrong too. Especially when it comes to long-term issues such as substance **abuse.**

Teens' knowledge about substance abuse is short-term. It may take several years for alcohol to cause serious physical harm and therefore cannot be something that teenagers know from their own personal experience. Nor do they always understand the damage it can do to family and work life.

And even if you assume, for argument's sake, that your friends know what's best for them, they may not know what's best for you.

You are a unique person, with your own needs, values, and goals. You have your own body, which may react differently to alcohol. You may have a family history of alcohol abuse, or you may have a family tradition of abstention (no alcohol); in either case, you may have good reasons to abstain, for now. Doing well on tomorrow's midterm exam may be a higher priority for you than for some of your friends; or maybe they are so smart they can ace the test even with a hang-over. Are you sure *you* can?

MANIPULATION BY PEERS

When friends talk, they should honestly say what is on their minds. Sometimes, however, even friends can have hidden agendas. In other words, they may try to manipulate you—make you do something you really did not want to do by telling you lies or only part of the truth.

Kids who drink or use illegal drugs may have several different reasons for manipulating you into joining them. They may feel they have protection in numbers: You might not tell on them if you're involved too. They may feel unsure that what they are doing is really safe, smart, or all that much fun; if they can convince you to join them, it may relieve their own doubts. And finally, misery loves company. Kids who are starting to feel the negative, harmful effects of alcohol abuse may not want to face them alone. Getting you into the same mess is not the best way to deal with their problem, but it may seem like a good idea to them.

Anyone who tries to manipulate you into doing something against your better judgment usually tries to play on your fears and emotional needs, including:

The fear of losing friends. You may be afraid of losing the friend who is manipulating you, or other friends, if you don't go along with his or her behavior.

The need to be popular, to be part of a crowd. You may not really want to drink, or to drink too much, but you may be willing to, if you think that's the price you have to pay to join a group. (But think of this: According to Minnesota prevention specialist Kris Van Hoof, "The easiest group to belong to is the users. They accept pretty much anybody. As long as you drink or use, you're in." Is that the group you *want* to belong to?)

The fear of looking like a geek. You may want to turn down alcohol simply because it doesn't make sense for you now. But if you don't drink, will people think you're a nerd? Don't wind up *doing* something stupid just to avoid *looking* stupid.

The fear of being different. If you think *everyone* does it, you may not have the strength to abstain.

The need to be polite. No one likes to hurt or insult their friends by turning down their offer of a drink. No one wants to seem "holier than thou."

The need for love and attention from the opposite sex. A friend may tell you that drinking makes you less shy, improves your sexual performance, or makes you more attractive. Even if you think that sounds off-base, you might *want* to believe it enough to try. If your friend really wants to manipulate you, he or she may offer you a drink in front of someone he or she knows you like. That is very tough to resist if the other person is drinking too.

It is also hard to resist when you happen to be feeling low, depressed, or anxious. You may be especially open to manipulation at times like those.

Q & A

Question: How can I turn down a drink from my best friend?

Answer: The easy answer is, you should be comfortable about being honest with a good friend: just say what you feel. But sometimes your friend might be insulted or annoyed anyway. If your values, not to say your health and safety, are important to you, you may just have to take that chance. If you have to face the same question over and over, maybe it's time for a serious talk—or time to seek out new friends.

RESISTING PEER PRESSURE

It is hard to say no to someone you like, but you may as well learn that skill while you are young. What words should you use? Whatever feels comfortable for you. Here are some lines that other kids have come up with. They won't all work every time, but they may inspire you to invent some lines of your own. Think it over *before* you get into a situation, so you are prepared when the time comes.

- Don't turn down your friend, just turn down the alcohol. For example, you might say, "I like hanging with you, but I just don't like getting drunk," or "We're friends, but we don't have to do everything together."
- Offer to do something else. "Let's go eat; let's go to a movie; let's call so-and-so." If your friends say no, tell them they can join up with you later.

- Give a good excuse. "I can't"; "I have to study tonight"; "I'm taking prescription drugs and I can't drink"; or "I'm in training" are always handy (provided they're true).

- Don't preach. This may not be the time for a real deep conversation. Just say, "It's cool, I just don't feel like it," or "I don't like the taste." You can make your point without putting down your friends.

- Turn it into a joke. "Sure, let's drink. Then when I total my car, maybe my dad will buy me a new one—if I'm still alive."

- Take time out. If you're at a party, for example, go to the bathroom or step outside to clear your head. Then, if they ask again, you'll probably feel strong enough to say what you really mean.

- If things are really getting out of hand, make yourself scarce. If you have a strong feeling you would rather be someplace else, go with it. You have a right to protect yourself; tomorrow you can tell your friends, "I had to get up early. You guys were out of it, so I just left."

- Say what adults say. When the waiter comes around and offers a refill, an adult might say, "I'm good, thanks," and cover his or her glass with a hand. Sounds cool, doesn't it? It *is* cool, since it's a way of taking control and doing what *you* want to do.

GIVE IT A TRY

Peer pressure, about drinking or any other subject, isn't easy to resist. But in the end, the chances are, you will wind up with more and better friends if you do what you think is right. It is certainly worth trying.

See also: Advertising and Counteradvertising Campaigns; Alcohol Abuse, The Risks of; Binge Drinking Among Teenagers; Underage Drinking

■ RECOVERY AND TREATMENT

Treating alcohol **abuse** (consequences of a drinking pattern that leads to intoxication or addiction causing behavioral problems) or alcoholism (a form of alcohol abuse in which the abuser is physically addicted to alcohol) can be a long, difficult process. Alcohol abusers often find that the hardest steps in the recovery process are the first ones: recognizing that they have a problem and deciding to fix it.

Many people who suffer from alcohol abuse do not want to admit that they are ill. Even when they do, they often hesitate to seek treatment, out of ignorance, fear, or a feeling of hopelessness. They are making a mistake. Alcohol abuse *can* be successfully treated. It takes time and effort, and there can be setbacks; but treatment has helped millions of alcoholics and alcohol abusers lead better lives.

Drinking can be unhealthy and dangerously habit-forming. You can—and should—avoid most of alcohol problems by learning sensible drinking behavior or by choosing to abstain (not drink at all). If you do not make a firm decision either way, you may find it very easy to fall into bad drinking habits—and very hard to pull yourself out.

Fact Or Fiction?

People can never recover from alcoholism.

The Facts: It is true that many people, including those who follow the philosophy of Alcoholics Anonymous, believe that recovery from alcohol abuse is a life-long task. But don't misunderstand what they are saying. Millions of people in all walks of life have successfully confronted their alcohol problems and changed their behaviors. They and their families and friends are living better lives, thanks to self-help or formal treatment.

Since the time 80 years ago when people first began to think of alcohol abuse as a disease rather than a moral failing, doctors and therapists have been looking for ways to cure or treat the sufferers. It is a complicated process, involving several different levels of treatment. First of all, doctors must treat the physical harm that alcohol has done to the abuser's body. Then, if the abuser wants to stop drinking, doctors or clinics must deal with the difficult and sometimes dangerous symptoms of **withdrawal.**

The most difficult aspect to treat is the behavior itself. Since alcohol abuse, or alcoholism, does not have one simple cause, doctors can not inoculate people with a vaccine to prevent it. Nor can they prescribe an antibiotic to cure the behavior. So many different physical, emotional, and social factors can contribute to alcohol abuse, and they combine in different ways in each individual. Each of these factors may need to be dealt with separately:

- physical cravings for alcohol
- emotional problems that make people vulnerable to addictive behavior
- family members, friends, or colleagues who drink a lot
- problems at home, school, or work that people may want to escape

Health-care professionals and self-help innovators use many different methods to treat these factors, with different degrees of success. Sometimes they argue among themselves about which method is best. They even disagree on the crucial question: How can one measure success in treating alcohol abuse?

With many diseases, such as measles or pneumonia, doctors try to cure the patients, to help them recover completely and return to good health. With other **chronic** (long-lasting) conditions, such as diabetes or **AIDS**, doctors today cannot cure the underlying problem. Instead, they try to keep the patients free of symptoms and help them to lead a normal life. Which kind of disease is alcohol abuse? Can anyone recover?

WHAT IS A RECOVERING ALCOHOLIC?

Nonaddictive alcohol abuse can sometimes be overcome by changes in lifestyle, such as a move or a new job. It is much harder, however, to deal with alcoholism itself. In fact, the majority of doctors and therapists practicing in the United States today believe that no one can ever completely recover from alcoholism.

A.A., or Alcoholics Anonymous, the largest and most influential self-help movement in the field, has been promoting that belief since it was founded in 1935. A.A. does accept that some "problem drinkers" may recover but believes that those who are truly alcoholic cannot. Most people under treatment for alcohol addiction are in programs inspired by A.A., and they are not aiming for complete recovery, or remission of symptoms. Instead, they call themselves **recovering alcoholics.**

According to A.A., recovery is an ongoing process that continues for the rest of the patient's life. A.A. members refer to themselves as alcoholics even years after their last drink of alcohol. They know that many nonalcoholics can handle moderate drinking, but they believe that a recovering alcoholic is always in danger of abusing alcohol again. They try to abstain from any form of alcohol. If they slip, as they sometimes do, they are committed to returning to **sobriety** (non-drinking). They also are committed to working on personal growth and helping other alcoholics and others in need.

Some treatment professionals do not agree that alcoholism is incurable. They believe that by dealing with the problems that contribute to addiction, and by learning new behaviors, alcoholics can be cured. Those experts define recovery as "a remission of symptoms over a certain period of time." In other words, the patient feels no cravings for alcohol for years at a time. The symptoms of abusive behavior may return in the future, like the symptoms of many other diseases. If they do, they can be treated once again.

Some individuals seem to recover without any formal treatment program. Sometimes a positive life change, such as a new job or the birth of a child, provides the incentive people need to face up to their drinking problem. And sometimes the opposite happens—a person realizes that alcohol is putting work, family, or even life itself at risk, and makes the decision to stop.

CAN THE ALCOHOLIC EVER DRINK SOCIALLY AGAIN?

This question has two parts. Experts disagree about the facts, but they also disagree about the message they want to convey to people who have not yet decided to seek treatment and to those who have been recovering for years.

Alcoholics Anonymous and the many other treatment programs it has inspired all give the question a firm answer: *no*. A.A.'s General Service Office writes, "All available medical testimony indicates that alcoholism is a progressive illness, that it cannot be cured in the ordinary sense of the term, but that it can be arrested through total abstinence from alcohol in any form." By progressive, they mean that the victims of this illness will always progress, or move along, from moderate drinking to addiction.

A.A. believes that alcoholics, by their very nature, have a tendency to abuse alcohol. Whether that tendency was inherited or learned from an alcoholic parent or acquired as a result of the ups and downs of life, A.A. believes that alcoholics are never able to get rid of their addiction completely.

A.A. advocates believe that the goal of abstinence is important, even if it is difficult to achieve. People may slip (by having a few drinks in a weak moment) or even have a relapse (by going back to problem drinking). But if they work toward abstinence as a goal, with the support of other A.A. members, the number and severity of their relapses can be limited.

Dr. Morris Chafetz, founding director of the National Institute for Alcohol Abuse and Alcoholism (NIAAA), wrote a book in 1976 called *Why Drinking Can Be Good for You*. As the title makes clear, he is not a prohibitionist, and he believes that many people's lives are improved by moderate drinking. However, he writes, "Social drinking after severe alcoholism isn't such a good idea." Even though statistics show that some alcoholics can carry it off, "why they'd run the risk is beyond me. Alcohol is no necessity of life."

Some critics of the A.A. philosophy would go further. They say that even alcoholics can eventually go back to social drinking. As evidence, they cite the National Longitudinal Alcoholism Epidemiological Survey, which was completed in 1992. The survey looked at several thousand people who had been alcohol-dependent 20 years before and divided them into two groups—those who had been in treatment programs and those who had not.

The survey came up with surprising results. Twenty years after people first became dependent on alcohol, more than half of those who never even sought treatment were now able to drink without abuse. On the other hand, only 25 percent of those who had undergone treatment could now drink socially.

Of course, it is usually the people suffering the most from alcohol who enter treatment—or are forced into treatment programs by family, employer, or judge. That may explain why those who were treated were less likely to overcome alcoholism. And many of those who say they can now drink socially may not have really been alcoholics.

The goal of total abstinence may frighten some people away from treatment. Those people are sometimes more willing to try programs that provide the option of cutting back rather than quitting. If that doesn't work, such patients are usually willing to try full abstinence.

FORMS OF TREATMENT

In 2007, there were 1.3 million people in the United States receiving treatment for alcohol abuse, according to the National Survey on Drug Use and Health. However, a much greater number, 18.1 million people,

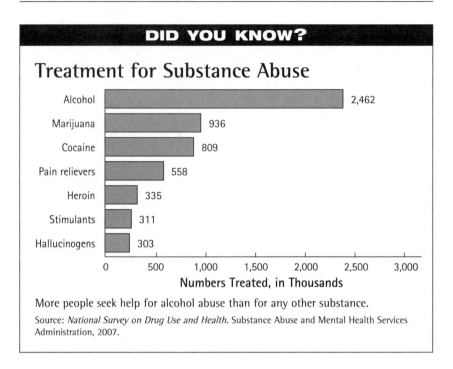

DID YOU KNOW?

Treatment for Substance Abuse

Substance	Numbers Treated, in Thousands
Alcohol	2,462
Marijuana	936
Cocaine	809
Pain relievers	558
Heroin	335
Stimulants	311
Hallucinogens	303

Numbers Treated, in Thousands

More people seek help for alcohol abuse than for any other substance.

Source: *National Survey on Drug Use and Health.* Substance Abuse and Mental Health Services Administration, 2007.

were classified as having some problem with alcohol dependence or alcohol abuse. Many different types of treatment are available. Some people use more than one of them over time, or even at the same time, to handle different aspects of their problems. The main variations are listed here.

Brief intervention

Brief intervention is a form of short-term therapy, aimed at changing behavior, that any trained social worker, educator, or physician can perform. In it, the professionals tell problem drinkers, or potential problem drinkers, about the risks they are facing and let them know how to reduce or eliminate the risks. Sometimes they refer people to treatment programs.

Some colleges use "feedback surveys" for brief intervention. They ask students to fill out questionnaires about their own drinking, and to estimate how much the average student drinks. When the results are tabulated and sent back to the participants, many students who drink much more than the average seem to reevaluate their behavior and cut back. World Health Organization researchers in Australia reported in 1994 that even five minutes of advice to problem drinkers leads many of them to cut back by 25 percent.

Psychotherapy

In psychotherapy, a psychologist, social worker, or other trained professional works with patients to help relieve their emotional or behavioral problems, usually through discussions or counseling sessions.

Among the popular forms of psychotherapy for alcoholics are:

- **Motivational enhancement therapy.** The therapist actively encourages the patient to consider the effects of alcohol on his or her life. Together, they create and put into effect a practical plan to reduce or eliminate drinking.

- **Cognitive behavior skills therapy.** Once patients figure out the specific "triggers" that make them want to have a drink (time of day, place, person, or situation), the therapist helps them find different ways to respond to those triggers without drinking. For example, the patient might learn to say no when someone offers them a drink, or to call a friend rather than go out for a drink when their boss chews them out at work.

- **Individual psychotherapy.** The patient tries to understand the underlying emotional reasons for his or her drinking behavior. This usually takes longer than other types of therapy.

- **Group therapy.** A group of patients meet to discuss each other's problems. This can help people learn to communicate better with others and give them greater self-confidence.

- **Social skills therapy.** The therapist focuses on improving the patient's interpersonal skills in the hope that he or she becomes more successful in work and social life. That success might make the patient less prone to seek out alcohol as an escape.

- **Stress management.** The patient is taught ways to deal with pressure without drinking, such as muscle relaxing, biofeedback, or meditation.

- **Family therapy.** The therapist meets with the patient's family and gets them involved in the treatment process.

Self-help programs

For more than 70 years, Alcoholics Anonymous (A.A.) has been help-ing millions of people around the world deal with alcohol abuse and lead better lives. It has developed a loyal following and has inspired other groups to use similar methods to deal with drug abuse and other addictions.

The famous A.A. **Twelve-Step program** leads members through a series of stages with the goal of becoming "recovering alcohol-ics." The steps are designed to encourage people to face up to their problem and to the damage it has caused themselves and others. The program relies on a great deal of mutual help among members and a commitment to help others in the community as well.

Q & A

Question: Is Alcoholics Anonymous (A.A.) a Christian organization?

Answer: The group does not define itself as religious, and it accepts people of all religious faiths—and even those who adhere to no reli-gion at all. Many present or former members say that critics of A.A. have exaggerated the religious aspect. However, the famous Twelve Steps does include several references to God "as we [each member] understands him." As a result, some people feel more comfortable attending other self-help groups that do not use the word *God*.

People who join and stick with A.A. share certain traits. They are more likely than the average alcoholic to have "hit bottom." They tend to be relatively extroverted, group-oriented, and able to discuss their problems with others. They also may be more religious and con-servative than others.

However, A.A. may not work for everyone. In recent years, several other self-help organizations have emerged, some of them founded by former A.A. members. If A.A. doesn't work for an individual alco-holic, he or she may be able to fit into one of these groups.

Institutional programs

Many private and government agencies offer programs that combine medical treatment, psychotherapy, and social work to help alcoholics deal with their problems. They are often based on the Minnesota Model, a recovery program that was developed at the Hazelden Foundation near Center City, Minnesota, in the 1960s.

The original program included 28-day inpatient (live-in) care, combining **detoxification** and medical help, clinical psychology, and after-care support. It followed A.A.'s Twelve-Step recovery philosophy, and like A.A., it used recovering alcoholics as counselors. The Betty Ford Clinic in California is another influential example of the Minnesota Model.

A similar idea is used by halfway houses. These facilities are designed for alcoholics who have gone through detoxification but are not fully prepared to resume their normal lives without alcohol. Residents work in their normal careers during the day and participate in treatment in the evenings. The period of treatment can range from a few weeks to several months.

Family life

Whatever their philosophy, professionals in the field of alcohol abuse all stress how important the patient's family is, both in contributing to alcohol abuse and in helping to overcome it. They encourage patients to involve their families in treatment whenever possible.

One method is family therapy, in which the patient and his or her spouse, parents, or children meet on a regular basis with a therapist. The goals are to help the family understand the patient's problems and to find ways they can help provide a healthier or more supportive atmosphere. In other programs, the therapist might meet separately with the patient's family.

Another method is the one followed by Al-Anon and Alateen, offshoots of Alcoholics Anonymous. Al-Anon members are relatives, or sometimes close friends, of alcoholics. They meet in small groups on a regular basis to discuss how to deal with an alcoholic family member. Their primary goal is to prevent the patient's alcohol problems from overwhelming the family. But they also examine some of their own behavior that may be keeping the patient from facing up to his or her problems. Alateen is a similar program, with membership restricted to teenage relatives and friends of alcoholics.

Other treatments

Some therapists and patients prefer treatments that put less emphasis on analyzing or changing the patient's frame of mind. Instead, they prefer shorter-term treatments that focus more attention on the patient's body.

"Natural recovery" has become popular in recent years. It tries to address the patient's overall health, nutrition, and lifestyle needs. Some common treatment techniques are acupuncture, yoga, biofeedback, and nutritional supplements.

In "Faradic" aversion therapy, doctors try to get alcoholics to hate alcohol by administering electric shocks while they drink or see pictures of alcoholic beverages.

Some doctors favor certain medications in treating alcohol, often in combination with other treatments:

- **Naltrexone** and other **antagonists** can be used to take away the "high" that comes with alcohol. These drugs attach themselves to the same nerve cells in the brain that alcohol uses, pushing alcohol aside until it can be broken down in the liver.

- **Aversion drugs** such as **Antabuse** make patients feel sick to their stomachs as soon as they drink any alcohol. These drugs condition some patients to dislike alcohol.

- Doctors often prescribe sedatives and antidepressants to help relieve the emotional symptoms that cause some people to drink too much.

WHAT ARE THE NUMBERS?

The field of alcohol treatment is large, diverse, and controversial. Many treatment programs publish statistics claiming certain recovery rates, but they rarely report long-term follow-ups. As a result, experts in the field cannot agree on any firm statistics. However, they all agree that treatment has helped millions of alcohol abusers.

In 2009, the authors of a study published in the *Journal of Studies on Alcohol and Drugs* reviewed the evidence on alcohol-treatment programs. They reported that treatment programs typically help reduce drinking and improve a person's quality of life.

In *The Facts About Drug Use* (A.A. Balkema, 1991) Barry Stimmel, a noted physician and medical educator specializing in addiction research, concedes that many people do not believe alcohol treatments work. But this "pessimism," he writes, "is unwarranted."

Stimmel compares alcoholism with diabetes or asthma, which are also **chronic** (long-term) diseases that cannot be fully cured. Doctors know, he writes, that most patients with those diseases *occasionally* eat improperly or occasionally fail to take their medicine, and many of them suffer relapses as a result. Yet no one wants to abandon diabetes or asthma patients or eliminate the treatment programs for those diseases. In the same way, alcohol abuse treatments should be judged on whether they improve the patient's quality of life over the *long haul*. It would be foolish to give up on alcoholism treatment programs just because many alcoholics occasionally slip up.

NO REASON TO LOSE HOPE

Alcoholism *can* be treated successfully. Millions of people testify to having overcome their dependence, using any of a wide variety of treatments. Alcohol abusers willing to explore the available treatment options, and then devote time and hard work, have every reason to expect recovery and a better life.

See also: Alcohol and Disease; Codependency; Peer Pressure and Alcohol; Screening for Alcoholism; Self-Help Programs; Withdrawal

FURTHER READING

Iliff, Brenda. *A Woman's Guide to Recovery.* Center City, Minn.: Hazelden, 2008.
Stimmel, Barry. *Alcoholism, Drug Addiction, and the Road to Recovery: Life on the Edge.* New York: Haworth Medical Press, 2002.

■ RISK TAKING

Behaviors that increase the probability of an unwanted event or potential loss. Elderly people know they may face health issues that are part of the normal aging process. Young people, in contrast, expect to enjoy robust good health, and most of them do. Unfortunately, some of them make behavior choices that put their health at risk. In fact, the major cause of death and chronic (long-term) illness among young people is risky behavior such as substance abuse, unsafe sex, and violence. That is why health educators try to focus on teenagers when dealing with risk taking.

In the 21st century, every American 15-year-old can expect to live another 65 years, at least. And most of those years should be healthy and productive. Of course, you never know what dangers beyond your control will come tomorrow. But you should know that behavior choices that are within your control can make a big difference in your chances of living a long and healthy life.

While young people like to experiment, even "push the envelope" now and then, risky habits formed in the teenage years can later be difficult to break. The right choices now may make your future healthier and, most likely, more successful and fulfilling.

Alcohol abuse is on every list of major risk-taking behaviors. In fact, drinking too much and combining drinking with driving or sexual behaviors are near the top of every risk-taking list.

THE CENTERS FOR DISEASE CONTROL AND PREVENTION

The Centers for Disease Control and Prevention, located in Atlanta, Georgia, is often in the headlines for its role in monitoring and controlling sudden epidemics and new viruses. But this federally funded institution also has responsibilities for preventing chronic disease, through its Center for Chronic Disease Prevention.

Concerned about risk taking among young people, the center set up the Youth Risk Behavior Surveillance System—YRBSS, for short—in 1990. By "surveillance," they weren't talking about spy satellites or telephone bugs. Instead, they have run repeated surveys, both nationwide and local, to ascertain how the country's teenagers were shaping up in terms of the following list of six major risk behaviors:

- Tobacco use
- Unhealthy dietary behaviors
- Inadequate physical activity
- Alcohol and other drug use
- Sexual behaviors that contribute to unintended pregnancy and sexually transmitted diseases, including HIV infection
- Behaviors that contribute to unintentional injuries and violence

These behaviors, the center said, were major contributors among teenagers to "the leading causes of death, disability, and social problems" (including heart disease, cancer, diabetes, and violent deaths). Furthermore, their reports show that the behaviors were "often established during childhood and early adolescence."

The center hoped that the surveys would uncover trends in young people's behavior, show the interconnections between different types of risk, highlight areas where education could improve behaviors, and monitor any improvements that education might bring.

YRBSS has conducted national, state, and local surveys of ninth- to 12th-grade youngsters every two years since 1991. The program also runs special surveys of college students, high-risk kids in alternative high schools, and surveys of the entire population of 12- to 20-year-olds. A number of promising state and local health education programs have grown out of these surveys. The results of the various YRBSS surveys are available online.

CONSEQUENCES

The YRBSS reports that for people between 10 and 24 years old, the leading causes of death in 2007 were

- Motor vehicle crashes: 25.6 per 100,000
- Homicide: 13.2 per 100,000
- Suicide: 9.7 per 100,000
- Other injury: 11.8 per 100,000
- HIV infection: 0.5 per 100,000
- All other causes: 12.3 per 100,000

Alcohol plays a role in many of these deaths. The 2007 YRBSS indicated that 29.1 percent of students had ridden at least once in a car with a driver who had been drinking alcohol in the past 30 days. More than 10 percent of students indicated they had driven a car with others when they had been drinking in the past 30 days. Nationwide, 4.1 percent of students admitted to drinking on school property in the past 30 days. Almost 24 percent (23.8) had started drinking alcohol before the age of 13. Alcohol also plays a role in sex, with 22.5 percent of sexually active students admitting to using either drugs or alcohol prior to sex.

ALTERNATIVES TO RISK TAKING

In life, you can't avoid taking *some* risks. Even if you could, it would be a boring life, especially for adventurous teenagers.

Educators concerned about unhealthy risk taking, however, have talked up the idea of *healthy* risk taking as an alternative. In her book

The Romance of Risk: Why Teenagers Do the Things They Do, adolescent psychotherapist Lynn Ponton suggests alternatives that might interest kids who are taking some dangerous risks. For example, kids involved in bullying or gang violence might want to take on the emotional risk of seeking out new friends or moving to a different school; those behaviors probably take a lot more courage than ganging up on a smaller kid.

As for alcohol- and drug-abusing teens, the book suggests that they look into the "extreme physical and emotional thrills" of whitewater rafting, rock climbing, and other vigorous sports. The key is to redefine "risk" as "challenge." What challenge do you meet, the writer asks, when you guzzle down five or six beers and jump behind the steering wheel?

Many schools around the United States and Canada have begun "alternatives to risk-taking" programs, built around after-school recreational, educational, and community service programs. Other schools have used that term as the title of class units that teach kids how to resist friends or classmates who try to pressure them into taking risks they do not want to take. Whichever alternatives they offer, these schools recognize that the old slogan "Just say no" may not be enough to convince today's kids.

BE SMART

Taking risks is part of life. Taking *harmful* risks when sensible alternatives are available is a part of life that smart teenagers avoid.

See also: Alcohol Abuse, The Risks of; Alcohol and Disease; Alcohol and Violence; Drinking and Driving; Effects on the Body; Sexual Behavior and Alcohol

FURTHER READING

Biglan, Anthony, Patricia A. Brennan, Sharon L. Foster, and Harold D. Holder. *Helping Adolescents at Risk: Prevention of Multiple Problem Behaviors.* New York: The Guilford Press, 2005.
Crouter, Ann C., and Alan Booth. *Romance and Sex in Adolescence and Emerging Adulthood: Risks and Opportunities.* Philadelphia: Lawrence Erlbaum Associates, 2005.
Kelsey, Candice M. *Generation MySpace: Helping Your Teen Survive Online Adolescence.* Cambridge, Mass.: Da Capo Press, 2007.

■ RISKS AND ALCOHOL

See: Alcohol Abuse, The Risks of

■ SCREENING FOR ALCOHOLISM

Tools used to determine if someone is addicted—physically and emotionally dependent upon—alcohol. It can be difficult to assess if someone occasionally drinks too much or has an alcohol problem, also known as alcohol use disorder. There are several different assessments that doctors have available. These include the ASSIST, MAST, AUDIT, CAGE, and other surveys. The assessments, often referred to as surveys, have proven to be quick and relatively accurate measures of alcohol use and alcoholism.

THE NEED FOR SCREENING TOOLS

The surveys are designed to enable health-care professionals to quickly determine if alcohol is a problem for someone. Because these surveys consist only of a few questions, however, the results are sometimes misleading, producing **false positive** or **false negative** test results. A false positive occurs when a person is screened and found to have an alcohol problem, even though one does not exist. A false negative occurs when a person is screened and found not to have a problem when one does exist.

Q & A

Question: What does it mean when someone talks about the "sensitivity" and "specificity" of a screening test?

Answer: *Sensitivity* refers to a survey's ability to properly identify people who have a disorder, which is an alcohol problem in this case. The fewer false negative cases there are, the greater the scale's "sensitivity."

Specificity refers to a survey's ability to identify people who do *not* have a disorder. The fewer false positives a survey produces, the greater its "specificity." No screening test will be 100 percent accurate; however, each type needs to be as close as possible in order to identify who needs help.

ALCOHOL, SMOKING AND SUBSTANCE INVOLVEMENT SCREENING TEST (ASSIST)

One of the screening tools used to assess an alcohol problem is the Alcohol, Smoking and Substance Involvement Screening Test. The ASSIST was developed by the World Health Organization (WHO) and an international team of substance-abuse researchers. The goal of the test is to screen people for problematic use of alcohol, tobacco, and other drugs, such as cocaine, opiates, and hallucinogens. The survey is designed to gather information about each of these substances. That can make this questionnaire time-consuming to complete, depending on how many substances a patient is thought to be using.

One of the first studies to use the ASSIST was published in 2002 in the journal *Addiction*. The authors tested the screening tool at treatment centers in several countries. The goal was to see how well the ASSIST worked. The results indicated that the ASSIST was a valid and reliable tool to measure problems with substance abuse. The survey was given to participants on two different occasions. Participants filled out the second survey between one and three days after completing the first survey. This was done to see if participants were consistent in their answers; it is referred to as a test-retest method of determining a survey's reliability.

A 2008 study in the journal *Addiction* was designed to see if the ASSIST test is a valid way to assess substance abuse problems. The authors of this study collected data from seven different countries, including Australia, Brazil, India, Thailand, England, Zimbabwe, and the United States. The data included the ASSIST measures as well as other measures of substance abuse. This allowed the authors to help determine if the ASSIST tool properly indicated if someone has a substance-abuse problem. The results indicate that the ASSIST survey is a valid measure of substance abuse. The survey can determine the level of someone's substance abuse as being of low, moderate, or high risk.

MICHIGAN ALCOHOLISM SCREENING TEST (MAST)

The Michigan Alcoholism Screening Test is another tool professionals use to help diagnose alcoholism. Unlike the ASSIST, the MAST focuses solely on alcohol problems. The survey contains 25 questions and asks about problems related to drinking, such as legal and medical consequences. It is designed to diagnose alcoholism, the addiction to alcohol. A score of zero to two indicates there is no drinking problem. A score between three and five indicates problems are starting, or have started, to develop (referred to as early to mid-stage problems). A score of six or greater is an indication of problem drinking.

The author of a 2001 study in the *Journal of Substance Abuse Treatment* evaluated the validity of the MAST. This was done by administering the test to people who had been repeatedly convicted of drunk driving. In addition to using the MAST, the Alcohol Use Disorders Identification Test (AUDIT) and the Diagnostic Criteria and Associated Questionnaire Items Test were employed. The authors found that the MAST is an effective tool to screen for alcohol problems.

Another study in a 2003 issue of *Addictive Behaviors* also focused on testing the validity of the MAST. The authors of this study collected data from people convicted of a DWI (driving while intoxicated) and people who had not been convicted of a DWI offense. The MAST was able to properly identify the three different groups in this study: nonoffenders, first-time offenders, and repeat offenders.

BRIEF MICHIGAN ALCOHOLISM SCREENING TEST

One of the problems with the MAST is its length. Twenty-five questions can be a lot to ask, especially in an emergency department of a hospital or in a doctor's office. To fix this problem, a shorter version of the survey was created—the bMAST.

The bMAST consists of the 10 "best" questions, which come from the MAST. Scores can range from zero to 29. A score of zero to four indicates there is no drinking problem. A score between five and 19 indicates there is the possibility of alcohol-related problems. A score of 20 or more indicates there is a high probability that the person being tested is dependent on alcohol.

A 2007 study in the *Journal of Studies on Alcohol and Drugs* provides evidence that the bMAST is a valid tool to assess the severity of problematic drinking. The authors studied two sets of data. One came from an alcohol-and-drug-treatment center, where the medical staff administered the bMAST and other screening tools. The second set of data also came from an alcohol-and-drug-treatment center. The difference is that at the second center, patients had also been asked an extensive series of questions from the *Diagnostic and Statistical Manual of Mental Disorders, Fourth Edition (DSM-IV)*. The patients met the *DSM-IV* criteria for alcohol problems, and the researchers were able to compare how well the bMAST correlated with the *DSM-IV* survey.

The authors also found that the bMAST was significantly correlated with the Alcohol Use Disorders Identification Test (AUDIT). This indicates that the bMAST is an accurate tool to assess the severity of alcohol dependence.

ALCOHOL USE DISORDERS IDENTIFICATION TEST (AUDIT)

Another screening test is the Alcohol Use Disorders Identification Test. This survey was also designed by the World Health Organization. There are 10 questions, and the survey was designed to be used in health-care settings to screen for dangerous drinking behavior. A score of eight or higher indicates harmful drinking behavior. For women, a score of 13 or higher indicates alcohol dependence, while men must score 15 or higher to indicate alcohol dependence.

The test identifies two aspects of alcohol misuse: alcohol consumption and alcohol-related consequences. The first three questions measure consumption of alcohol. Four other questions focus on the consequences of alcohol use.

A 2007 study in the journal *Drug and Alcohol Dependence* validates the AUDIT. The authors of this study examined a modified version of the AUDIT. The questions were asked over the telephone as part of a larger study on alcohol.

The authors of a 2007 study in *Alcoholism: Clinical and Experimental Research* reviewed five years of research on the AUDIT. Their goal was to assess the overall effectiveness of AUDIT in various settings and groups, such as racial and ethnic groups, adolescents, women, and patients with other medical or mental-health issues in addition to drinking problems. Results indicated that the AUDIT is an accurate tool to screen for alcohol use disorders.

ALCOHOL USE DISORDERS IDENTIFICATION TEST—CONSUMPTION (AUDIT-C)

The AUDIT-C is a three-item test, with the questions coming from the longer AUDIT. This brief test assesses risky drinking problems by asking questions on alcohol consumption. The score can range from zero to 12, with a score of three or more indicating problematic alcohol consumption in women. A score of four or more indicates problematic alcohol consumption in men.

Findings from a 2008 study in the *Journal of General Internal Medicine* indicate that the AUDIT-C is an excellent measure of "risky drinking." In this study, the authors also examined the test's ability to measure alcohol misuse in both men and women and in three racial groups (whites, Hispanics, and African Americans). Although the AUDIT-C proved to work well for men and women in all three racial groups, the test had the strongest sensitivity for Hispanic women and white men. Conversely, the lowest sensitivity was for African-American men and women.

This means that although the AUDIT-C is, overall, an accurate measure of alcohol misuse, it simply works better for some groups than others.

CUT-ANNOYED-GUILT-EYE QUESTIONNAIRE (CAGE)

The Cut-Annoyed-Guilt-Eye questionnaire is a four-question screening tool also used to assess alcohol problems. The questions are very simple:

Have you ever felt you should cut down on your drinking?

Have people annoyed you by criticizing your drinking?

Have you ever felt bad or guilty about your drinking?

Have you ever had a drink first thing in the morning to steady your nerves or get rid of a hangover (an eye-opener)?

The answers are all yes/no. People who answer "yes" to two or more questions are said to have a problem with their drinking.

The authors of a 2009 study in the *Journal of Psychosomatic Research* examined the relationship between problems with alcohol and death (from all causes). To assess alcohol problems, the CAGE was used. The results indicated that people with alcohol problems were at a higher risk of dying than those without drinking problems.

Although the CAGE was first published in 1984, few doctors have heard of it. The author of a 2008 article in the *Journal of the American Medical Association* reviewed evidence on the use of the CAGE by doctors. According to the author, only about 50 percent of doctors have heard of the CAGE. Worse, the author provided evidence that only 30 percent of primary-care physicians even screen for alcohol problems in their practice. Of these doctors, only 55 percent use the CAGE.

Researchers and medical experts agree that the younger a child is when he or she starts to drink, the more likely he or she is to develop drinking problems and become dependent on alcohol. Yet, many doctors do not routinely test for signs of alcoholism. Given the effectiveness and simplicity of a screening test such as the four-question CAGE, for example, the authors of the 2008 article in the *Journal of the American Medical Association* believe that more doctors must incorporate these valuable tools into their practices.

See also: Alcoholism, Causes of; Drinking and Driving

FURTHER READING
Mignon, Sylvia, and Peter L. Myers. *Substance Use and Abuse: Exploring Alcohol and Drug Issues.* Boulder, Colo.: Lynne Rienner Publishers, 2009.

■ SELF-HELP PROGRAMS

A series of steps or services that help overcome a problem. Alcohol abuse can be a very sad topic, but one inspiring chapter in the story is the self-help movement created by alcoholics and their families. Through hard work, courage, and initiative, they have developed new ways of dealing with alcoholism and other addictive behaviors. They have given new hope and confidence to millions of people.

HISTORY OF ALCOHOLICS ANONYMOUS

The story of A.A., or Alcoholics Anonymous, began in Akron, Ohio, in 1935. The founders were "Bill W.," a stockbroker, and "Dr. Bob S.," a surgeon, both of whom had been severe alcoholics.

Bill had become sober through his membership in the Oxford Group, a Christian organization that tried to bring spiritual values into daily life. Some of the techniques of A.A., and much of its Twelve-Step philosophy came from the Oxford Group. But the core idea that alcoholism should be considered a disease came from Dr. William Silkworth, a physician to whom Bill had often gone for detoxification treatment.

The two founders, Bill W. and Dr. Bob, decided early on that only alcoholics themselves could help one another overcome their specific problems. They spread their message among other alcoholics and helped organize groups of like-minded alcoholics into small self-help groups. By 1939, when Bill published *Alcoholics Anonymous,* a book-length guide to recovery with successful case histories, about 100 members had become sober in three different cities.

The group filled a desperate need for treatment; its message of hope proved appealing. A.A. has not stopped growing since. By 1951, a "General Service Conference" was formed to provide central services and publish books and pamphlets for members of the groups and interested outsiders.

In 1939, family groups began to form as an outgrowth of A.A. Relatives of alcoholics got together to discuss the problems that alcoholism brings to the families and friends of alcoholics. In 1951, Bill W.'s wife cofounded Al-Anon to coordinate the several dozen groups that had formed in the United States and abroad. By 1997, Al-Anon Family Groups, the coordinating body, claimed that 30,000 groups exist in 115 countries.

Alateen, devoted to teenage family members and friends of alcoholics, was founded in 1957. Like Al-Anon, it adheres to the Twelve-Step philosophy, and its groups function in accordance with the A.A. model.

A.A. TODAY

Alcoholics Anonymous, the pioneer organization in treating alcohol abuse, now claims more than one million members in the United States, organized into more than 50,000 self-supporting local groups. A.A.'s affiliates (associated groups) around the world have another million members. Millions of past members have also recovered in whole or in part as a result of A.A.

According to a 2007 membership survey (published by the A.A. General Service Conference), men outnumber women by 67 percent to 33 percent. All age groups are represented, though only one out of nine members is under 30 years old. More than one-third are married, another third are single, and about one-quarter are divorced. The group is racially and economically diverse, although a large majority of members are whites.

The average member attends two meetings a week. Most important, the survey reports that members have been sober for an average of seven years. The large majority of members have also taken advantage of other forms of treatment or counseling, often while attending A.A. group meetings.

The group describes itself as "a fellowship of men and women who share their experience, strength and hope with each other that they may solve their common problem and help others to recover from alcoholism." Members run and fund their own groups, along guidelines provided by the national organization. Membership is free, and tradition ensures that anyone who wants to become sober is welcomed.

A.A. has continued its practice of strict anonymity—people are known on a first-name basis only—even though alcoholism is no longer considered shameful by most people. In today's world, A.A. says, anonymity helps to keep the organization free of power struggles and corruption. Any group leadership positions are rotated among the members.

The basic treatment philosophy of A.A. is that "an alcoholic who no longer drinks has an exceptional faculty for 'reaching' and helping an uncontrolled drinker." In others words, the best person to help an alcoholic recover is a recovering alcoholic. Toward that end, the group aims to provide a "sponsor" to each new member. The sponsor is available at all times to share his or her experiences, provide moral support, and help the "sponsee" overcome any problems that could lead him or her back to alcohol abuse. The 2007 survey found that 79 percent of members had a sponsor and that 73 percent had gotten a sponsor within 90 days of joining up.

Members are supposed to be guided by the "Twelve Steps" to recovery. The first step, which is said to be the most difficult, is for alcoholics to admit that they are "powerless over alcohol." In other words, they cannot beat the problem without help from a "Power greater than ourselves," which A.A. defines as "God as we understand Him."

Several steps revolve around members taking a "moral inventory," trying to understand their faults and the way they have hurt other people. They then try to "make amends" with the people they have harmed. Finally, they make a commitment to spread the message to other alcoholics and to conduct themselves according to these principles in the future.

Someone who decides to try A.A., or has been sent to A.A. by a treatment program, usually attends orientation meetings, aided by a guide who sometimes becomes the sponsor. The new member is then encouraged to make a commitment to attend a certain number of meetings, often 90 meetings in 90 days, even if they must put aside

The Twelve Steps

Alcoholics Anonymous recommends the Twelve Steps listed below as a guide for individuals trying to overcome alcoholism. Many other self-help groups now use similar steps in their recovery programs.

1. We admitted we were powerless over alcohol—that our lives had become unmanageable.

2. Came to believe that a Power greater than ourselves could restore us to sanity.

3. Made a decision to turn our will and our lives over to the care of God as we understood Him.

4. Made a searching and fearless moral inventory of ourselves.

5. Admitted to God, to ourselves and to another human being the exact nature of our wrongs.

6. Were entirely ready to have God remove all these defects of character.

7. Humbly asked Him to remove our shortcomings.

8. Made a list of all persons we had harmed, and became willing to make amends to them all.

9. Made direct amends to such people wherever possible, except when to do so would injure them or others.

10. Continued to take personal inventory and when we were wrong promptly admitted it.

11. Sought through prayer and meditation to improve our conscious contact with God, as we understood Him, praying only for knowledge of His will for us and the power to carry that out.

12. Having had a spiritual awakening as the result of these steps, we tried to carry this message to alcoholics and to practice these principles in all our affairs.

other personal commitments to do so. In most cities, there are groups meeting every day.

Even for those who find the meetings helpful, it may take some time before a new member admits to having a problem and makes the famous statement, "My name is ––, and I am an alcoholic." In fact, the earliest stage is probably crucial to success within the group. Success seems to depend in part on how accepting the group is.

Many A.A. members are firmly convinced that they would not have been able to overcome their problems without A.A. The acceptance and support they get from other members made it easier for them to adopt new ways of thinking about themselves and new, more healthy behaviors.

A.A., however, is not necessarily the best treatment for every individual. People who attend a few meetings and drop out should not consider themselves failures. It may be that another A.A. group, or a different self-help program, or another type of treatment altogether, may be more to their liking. Besides, even "dropouts" can benefit from the stories they hear and the literature they read while attending A.A.

AL-ANON

Al-Anon was founded by family members of A.A. members, and follows A.A.'s Twelve-Step philosophy; however, the two groups are not formally connected, and Al-Anon is run independently both on the local and national levels.

Al-Anon members consider alcoholism to be a "family disease." When one member of a family is a serious alcoholic, everyone else suffers to a degree. Families often may be harmed in practical ways, when the alcoholic fails to carry his or her weight financially or as a good spouse or parent. Sometimes the emotional toll is even higher, with fear, anger, resentment, and loneliness taking over the home.

Too often, family members also may be victimized by violence at the hands of the alcoholic individual. Members are encouraged to learn how to protect themselves and, if necessary, to involve the authorities. Al-Anon believes that no one is helped when families try to protect violent alcoholics from the consequences of their behavior.

The purpose of Al-Anon is to allow members to help one another by sharing their stories and successes in dealing with their common problems. They believe this process helps them change their own unhealthy attitudes and behaviors that result from their relative or friend's alcoholism.

Al-Anon believes that the alcoholic must work towards his or her own recovery. But the family can help avoid behaviors that "enable" the alcoholic to remain stuck in his or her disease. For example, they must stop making excuses for the alcoholic and must look out for the family's interest even at the expense of the alcoholic, if he or she is uncooperative.

Some 85 percent of Al-Anon members are women, most often the wives of alcoholics. They tend to be a bit older than the average A.A. member but otherwise represent a cross-section of people. Their alcoholic family member is not necessarily a member of A.A., and may not even be in treatment. In fact, Al-Anon's literature insists that "no situation is really hopeless and that it is possible to find contentment and even happiness, whether the alcoholic is drinking or not."

As is the case with A.A., the majority of Al-Anon members have participated in other counseling or treatment programs to help deal with their family's alcoholism problems. Al-Anon meetings help reinforce the benefits of those programs.

ALATEEN

Teenagers with an alcoholic family member (who is usually a parent) experience all the problems of other family members, and perhaps a few more of their own. Adolescents should be able to rely on parents for advice and support as they learn to become adults. Instead, many teen children of alcoholics get little or no support from the alcoholic parent. They often get less support than they need even from the nonalcoholic parent, who may be preoccupied.

Kids tend to care very much about what their friends and schoolmates think. Frequently embarrassed by their alcoholic parent's behavior, they may even withdraw from friends; angry or frustrated, they sometimes misbehave in and out of school.

Alateen, like its parent-group Al-Anon, takes many of its ideas from A.A., including anonymity, the Twelve Steps, sponsors, and the idea of mutual help among people sharing the same problems. Every Alateen group has an adult sponsor who is a member of Al-Anon.

There are now some 24,000 Alateen groups meeting around the world. The average age of members is 14; 65 percent are girls.

OTHER SELF-HELP GROUPS

Over the years, former members of A.A. who felt that the organization did not meet their particular needs, and other people who disagreed with parts of the A.A. philosophy, have created several other types of self-help groups. None of them has grown nearly as large as A.A., but they can be a useful alternative for some people.

Women for Sobriety was founded in 1976, when the modern feminist movement was in full swing. Its members believe that women's recovery needs are different from men's and are not fully recognized by A.A. They agree with A.A.'s disease model of alcoholism and its goal of **abstinence,** and like A.A. their "New Life" program includes a system of levels (steps) and statements of principles. But they stress individual responsibility for change rather than reliance on a "higher power." The group boasts several hundred groups in six countries.

Secular Organizations for Sobriety has been in existence since 1986. It is designed "for those alcoholics or drug addicts who are uncomfortable with the spiritual content" of A.A. and similar groups. They claim member groups in every state and some foreign countries. Like A.A., they advocate abstinence.

SMART (Self Management and Recovery Training, founded in 1994) is another nonspiritual self-help organization with a few hundred member groups. It rejects the disease model of alcoholism and does not advocate lifetime membership. They offer online groups as well.

Moderation Management was founded in 1993. It is the only alcoholism self-help organization that believes in moderate drinking as a possible goal—but only after the new member goes through a period of abstinence. It is designed for "problem drinkers" rather than alcoholics, especially drinkers in the "beginning stage" who have not progressed to serious alcohol **dependency.**

FROM PAIN TO INSPIRATION

Thanks to the success of Alcoholics Anonymous, self-help groups have proliferated (spread widely) in communities all across the United States. Together they offer information, encouragement, and inspiration to millions of people.

See also: Children of Alcoholics; Ethnicity and Alcohol; Law and Drinking, The; Recovery and Treatment

FURTHER READING

Alcoholics Anonymous World Services. *Alcoholics Anonymous: The Story of How Many Thousands of Men and Women Have Recovered from Alcoholism.* New York: Alcoholics Anonymous World Services, 2001.

Nowinski, Joseph. *The Twelve-Step Facilitation Handbook: A Systematic Approach to Early Recovery from Alcoholism and Addiction.* San Francisco, Calif.: Jossey-Bass, 1998.

Prentiss, Chris. *The Alcoholism and Addiction Cure: A Holistic Approach to Total Recovery.* Malibu, Calif.: Power Press, 2007.

Trapani, Margi. *Inside a Support Group: Help for Teenage Children of Alcoholics.* New York: Rosen Publishing Group, 1997.

■ SEXUAL BEHAVIOR AND ALCOHOL

Drinking and sex have one thing in common. They can be safe when done wisely and carefully. But if you do either one foolishly, you can get into trouble. And if you do them foolishly at the same time, you double your risk.

Drinking and sex are connected in another way. Some people deliberately use alcohol to overcome shyness and initiate social or sexual contact with an appropriate partner. Others believe that alcohol increases their sexual drive or performance or at least makes them feel more relaxed and able to respond to their partner.

Combining sex and alcohol has a big negative side too. Alcohol may lead many people to give in to sex when they really want to say no. Sex and alcohol also may lead to unwanted pregnancy, **sexually transmitted diseases (STDs)**, violence, and rape, and can cause guilt, fear, and broken relationships. The problem is separating the good from the bad.

IS ALCOHOL AN APHRODISIAC?

According to research, **aphrodisiacs** (foods or drinks that increase romantic or sexual desire) do not really exist, although you could spend a bundle on the Internet buying products that promise to do the trick. Yet for many people, one or two drinks have a relaxing effect, distracting them from their worries and loosening the control centers in their brains. As a result, they may feel more tender and loving, at the right time and place, and more aware of their natural sexual feelings.

On the other hand, as people continue drinking, the opposite effect kicks in. Sex involves two people, and therefore needs sensitivity and attention, which usually go out the window when people are intoxicated. And if you keep on drinking, you can become unable to perform—even if you can stay awake. As one expert put it, "Heavy drinkers have lousy sex lives."

Alcohol can stimulate sex in another, more sinister, way. Some people believe that alcohol makes them more virile and desirable. Since they are often mistaken, this belief can lead to misunderstandings and even serious trouble for others.

Fact Or Fiction?

Alcohol can improve a man's sexual performance.

The Facts: This one is somewhat true, but mostly false. A small amount of alcohol may help some men relax and feel sociable, which is helpful in any kind of romantic or sexual situation. But if a man has several drinks, his ability to do any physical task, including sex, starts to decline rapidly. Habitual heavy drinking can lead to impotence and even sterility.

SEXUAL COERCION

Sexual coercion, in which one person forces another person to have sexual relations against his or her will, can take many forms. Its most extreme form is rape, in which one person forces the other to have sexual relations against his or her will.

Rape is a violent crime that is rightly punished by long prison sentences. It can inflict terrible emotional damage on its victims, as well as serious practical consequences such as unwanted pregnancy (a woman carrying the rapist's child) or sexually transmitted disease. Alcohol use is strongly connected with rape, both statistically (a high percentage of rapists drink before the rape) and psychologically (alcohol may "prepare" the rapist for the crime).

According to the authors of a 2009 study in *Addictive Behaviors*, the evidence suggests that approximately 50 percent of sexual assault offenders had been drinking prior to or during the assault. The authors also found that those who drink heavily are more likely to misinterpret someone's sexual intentions, were more forceful, and

DID YOU KNOW?

Role of Alcohol in Crimes of Violence

Perceived drug or alcohol use by offender	Crimes of violence	Rape/ Sexual Assault	Robbery	Percent of victimizations Total	Assault Aggravated	Simple
Total victimizations	100.0%	100.0%	100.0%	100.0%	100.0%	100.0%
Total (Perceived to be under the influence of drugs or alcohol)	27.1	42.8	24.8	26.6	27.0	26.5
Under the influence of alcohol	15.2	26.8	12.4	15.0	14.5	15.1
Under the influence of drugs	5.6	1.2*	7.1	5.6	5.2	5.7
Under the influence of both drugs and alcohol	5.2	14.8	5.1*	4.8	5.8	4.4
Under the influence of one, not sure which	1.0	0.0*	0.0*	1.2	1.5*	1.2
Not available whether drugs or alcohol	0.1*	0.0*	0.2*	0.0*	0.0*	0.0*
Not on alcohol or drugs	27.0	19.0	14.1	29.2	24.0	31.0
Don't know or not ascertained	45.9	38.2	61.1	44.2	49.0	42.5

*Estimate based on 10 or fewer sample cases

Alcohol and drugs play a significant role in violent crimes. This is especially noticeable for rapes and sexual assaults, including threats of those crimes.

National Crime Victimization Survey. Bureau of Justice Statistics, 2006.

committed more severe assaults. Authors of another study, published in 2009 in *Addictive Behaviors,* found that female alcohol and drug use during an assault is a risk factor for rape.

It is not surprising that many victims of sexual coercion have been drinking themselves. Women become intoxicated more quickly after drinking the same amount of alcohol as a man. Once intoxicated, they may miss warning signs that they are in danger and once they do understand, they may be unable to communicate their disapproval forcefully enough.

When sexual attacks begin, victims who have been drinking may not have the mental and physical resources they need to fight off their attackers. After the rape is over, they may feel shame that they drank enough to put themselves in danger, or they may not remember enough of the details to be sure of what really happened. But when victims regret their own actions, it does not excuse the rapist or the crime. It only highlights that taking advantage of someone against her will is a cowardly act as well as a criminal one.

Acquaintance rape, where the victim knew the perpetrator before the attack took place, is often associated with alcohol. On college campuses, according to a 2001 Justice Department report, nearly 90 percent of victims of rape or attempted rape on campuses personally knew the offender. In most of those, both the attacker and the victim had been drinking.

UNINTENDED SEX

People change their minds all the time, about sex as much as any other thing. Two "consenting adults" might have every intention of engaging in sexual relations on a particular occasion, yet something gets in the way (for example, drinking too much), and the plans fall through. But in other cases, one or both of the parties may have no intention of having sex, but under the influence of alcohol they change their minds.

It is not surprising that alcohol, the original "disinhibitor" that allows people to do things they wouldn't do sober, can lead to unplanned sex. A 2002 study by the Kaiser Family Foundation found that 29 percent of people between 15 and 17 years old admit that they are more sexually active than they plan to be due to alcohol and drug use. The number rises to 37 percent for the 18 to 24 age group.

A 1999 college survey reported by the Harvard University School of Public Health found that binge drinkers (men who drink five or more alcoholic drinks at one time, and women who drink four or more) were five times more likely to have unplanned sex as other students.

Unintended sex is usually unprepared and unprotected sex as well. It is often unappreciated too, the morning after. When sober, most people say that sex is important enough for them to carefully choose the time, place, and partner ahead of time. Under the influence of alcohol, however, people are less likely to stick to their own standards.

UNPROTECTED SEX

To state the obvious: Sex can have serious consequences. A woman of childbearing age (usually from the teenage through the middle-age years) is at risk of becoming pregnant from a single, brief sexual encounter, unless she or her partner deliberately uses birth control. Also, anyone who is careless about sex is at risk of getting a sexually transmitted disease, no matter what type of sexual behavior is involved.

Common sense suggests that people who are drinking when they have sex are less likely to use protection, since alcohol weakens the rational control centers of the brain. However, the evidence from surveys is not clear. One study published in 2003 in the journal *Perspectives on Sexual and Reproductive Health* found that teens were just as likely to use condoms after drinking alcohol than when they have not been drinking. However, other studies show that men and women who drink and also use drugs are much less likely than others to use condoms during sex. In those cases, it is hard to prove that alcohol is the cause of unprotected sex. A careless disregard for risk may cause both behaviors.

Unwanted pregnancies

As everyone knows, the only guaranteed way to avoid unwanted pregnancy is to abstain from sex. If you choose to practice **abstinence** before marriage, remember that it is easier to stick with your principles if you remain sober. The more you drink, the less likely you are to remain true to your values.

The next most effective methods available to women to keep from becoming pregnant are birth control pills, shots, patches, or skin implants, which prevent ovulation (the release of eggs in the womb), and intrauterine devices (IUD), which block sperm from reaching the egg. None of these methods requires protective action at the time of sex, so alcohol does not increase the risk of pregnancy.

Many women, especially young women, rely on condoms as their first line of defense—which means they must rely on men to use condoms too. To be fully effective, condoms have to be used correctly. For example, people should only use unopened condoms from an unbroken package that has not passed its expiration date. They should not use any petroleum-based lubricant, such as Vaseline, which can break down the latex in the condom. They should leave room at the tip of the condom to collect semen and keep it from seeping out the top. They should keep the condom on after withdrawal, and they should throw it away after use. Also, according to most experts, they should use latex rather than lambskin condoms to protect against sexually transmitted diseases (STDs), although both types are equally effective in preventing pregnancy. Now, do you think you can remember and carry out all these instructions after having several drinks?

Sexually transmitted diseases (STDs)

Until the invention of antibiotics early in the 20th century, STDs were recognized as a very serious threat to public health (they were called "venereal diseases" in those days). Syphilis, perhaps the most feared of the STDs, often led to insanity and death.

The introduction of penicillin in the 1940s seemed to promise a world free of STDs. Before too long, however, the bacteria and other organisms that cause the most common STDs started developing resistance to penicillin and other antibiotic drugs. Today, it takes larger and larger doses of antibiotics to knock out a syphilis or gonorrhea infection. Even worse, the medical profession soon learned that serious virus infections, such as herpes and hepatitis B and C, were being widely spread through sexual contact.

The list of common STDs has grown with time. The world has become a smaller place; tiny disease-bearing organisms from all over the world seem to travel as easily as the most restless jet setter. The list includes chlamydia (which can cause sterility), fungus infections, yeast infections, venereal lice, and human papilloma virus (which can cause cervical cancer).

In 1981, a new STD surfaced—acquired immunodeficiency syndrome, or **AIDS**. Though it can also be passed from one person to another through contact with infected blood, most patients have been infected during sexual activity.

Every year about 19 million new cases of STDs occur in the United States. The two main risk factors that help spread STDs so widely are unprotected sex and multiple sexual partners.

Unprotected sex allows the exchange of infected body fluids, like semen or traces of blood. An infected individual may have enough bacteria or virus particles in those body fluids to infect the healthy partner after just one sexual contact. This is possible even if the infected partner does not show any symptoms of the disease. Almost any type of sexual activity between unprotected partners has the potential of spreading STDs.

The chances of transmission are increased if either partner has a sore or skin infection to begin with, or if his or her skin is chafed or torn during sex. The risk of transmission during unprotected sex is 30 percent for herpes, and up to 50 percent for gonorrhea.

The most effective protection against STDs during sex is a latex condom. Other birth control methods, such as pills, IUDs, diaphragms, and spermicidal creams, do nothing to protect against STDs. Lambskin condoms have tiny holes big enough for HIV, the virus that causes AIDS, to pass through.

Since alcohol can impair people's judgment and self-control, people who have been drinking often neglect to use condoms or fail to use them properly. Alcohol may play an even greater role in the other major risk factor for STDs—multiple sex partners.

According to a 2008 report by the New York City Department of Health and Mental Hygiene, 27 percent of teens who drank alcohol in the past 30 days had multiple sex partners, compared to 11 percent of teens who did not drink. Sixty-three percent of teens who drank used a condom during sex, while 72 percent of nondrinking teens used a condom.

Q & A

Question: Do I need to practice safe sex if my partner has never had sex before?

Answer: If both you *and* your partner have never had sex of any kind with any other person, you will both remain free of STDs. But anyone who agrees to have sex with you may have agreed to have sex with another person. In other words, it really makes sense to play it safe— don't let alcohol cloud your judgment: Abstain from sex or limit your partners, and *practice safe sex every time*.

HIV and AIDS

In 1981, doctors in several American cities detected an epidemic of a new disease they named AIDS, or Acquired Immunodeficiency Disease. Two years later researchers discovered the organism that caused the disease—the human immunodeficiency virus (HIV)—and they showed that it could be easily passed along during sexual contact.

People can get infected with HIV through other means as well, such as sharing hypodermic needles or getting a transfusion of infected blood, but the large majority of victims have acquired the virus during sexual activity. If one unprotected partner has HIV, the other has a 1–4 percent chance of getting the virus during each sexual act. The risk depends on the particular act they perform.

HIV does its damage by harming, and eventually destroying, the body's immune system. This process can take several years to develop, but once the immune system is damaged the body becomes more vulnerable to dangerous and fatal illnesses such as pneumonia, painful nerve inflammations, liver disease, and cancer. By 2002, according to the Centers for Disease Control, AIDS had killed 501,000 Americans.

It took some 15 years before drugs were developed that could control AIDS. Drugs discovered in the 1990s have been successful in holding off fatal complications in most patients, and AIDS deaths began to decline in the United States. But these drugs are expensive, and they have not been available for most AIDS victims in poor countries. In 2007, according to the Joint United Nations Program on HIV/AIDS, more than 2 million people in countries all over the world died of AIDS. Some 2.5 million new people were infected with HIV in 2007.

New strains of HIV have begun to appear that the medicines cannot reach. In any case, these drugs only help people who are already sick; so far, no one has been able to make a vaccine that can be given to healthy people to keep the virus away.

When the epidemic first broke out in the United States, most of the victims were gay (homosexual) men. That has changed a long time ago, as the virus spread into wider communities. In most of the world, most people with AIDS are straight (heterosexual), and about half are women.

Due to the rise of AIDS, unprotected sex is far more dangerous than ever before. There has never been a better reason to use a latex condom. This is true for heterosexuals as well as for homosexuals. It is just as true for women and girls as for men and boys. It does not matter what part of the country you come from, what neighborhood you live in, or what race or ethnic group you belong to.

The best way to keep free of HIV is to abstain from sex. The next best way is to practice safe sex. That means you should:

- use good judgment in choosing sex partners;
- keep the number of partners to a minimum;

- avoid any activity that might cause skin tears or abrasions; and

- always use a condom, no matter what act you perform.

This is where alcohol comes in. Alcohol, especially in large quantities, can influence people to break every one of the rules of safe sex. It can lead you to have sex when you did not intend to or do not even want to; it impairs your judgment in choosing a partner; a pattern of alcohol abuse can lead to multiple partners; the lack of mental control can cause you to "forget" to use a condom; and the lack of physical control could make skin tears and abrasions more likely.

A study at Louisiana State University in 2003 suggested an even more direct link between alcohol and HIV. When alcohol is present in the bloodstream, researchers found, the body may be more susceptible to being infected by HIV during sexual contact.

Everyone knows that kids can make mistakes. It is part of growing up. But getting AIDS is too high a price to pay for the mistake of carelessly mixing drink and sex. Wouldn't you agree?

A DANGEROUS MIX

Drinking and driving is such a dangerous combination that it is against the law. Drinking and sex is not against the law, but don't be fooled—it can be very dangerous too.

Mature, experienced adults can usually handle the risks. Teenagers experimenting with these powerful behaviors very often can't. Smart kids do not allow social pressure and opportunity to take them down this path before they are ready. What's the rush?

See also: Alcohol and Violence; Binge Drinking Among Teenagers; Drinking on College Campuses; Risk Taking

FURTHER READING

Brynie, Faith Hickman. *101 Questions About Sex and Sexuality.* Brookfield, Conn.: Twenty-First Century Books, 2003.

Gerdes, Louise I. *Sexual Violence.* Opposing Viewpoints. Farmington Hills, Mich.: Greenhaven Press, 2008.

Wiesz, Arlene N., and Beverly M. Black. *Programs to Reduce Teen Dating Violence and Sexual Assault: Perspectives on What Works.* New York: Columbia University Press, 2009.

■ TAKING RISKS
See: Risk Taking

■ TEENAGERS AND ALCOHOL
See: Binge Drinking Among Teenagers; Children of Alcoholics; Choices, Responsible; Drinking and Driving; Peer Pressure and Alcohol; Underage Drinking

■ TOLERANCE AND REVERSE TOLERANCE
Body's ability to adjust to the effects of alcohol. Tolerance is a sign that the body is becoming accustomed to the presence of alcohol. When people develop tolerance to alcohol, their bodies need more alcohol to produce the desired effects, such as feeling a buzz or becoming intoxicated. However, it is also possible to develop reverse tolerance. This happens when the liver is damaged from chronic alcohol intake. Because the liver is not functioning properly, it cannot **metabolize**, or break down, the alcohol as it should. In turn, a person can get drunk easier than in the past.

Tolerance and reverse tolerance also increase the hazards of all the undesired effects of being drunk. There is often a fine line between tolerance and dependence, where individuals are so accustomed to drinking that they cannot function without it.

TYPES OF TOLERANCE
According to the National Institute on Alcohol Abuse and Alcoholism, there are several types of alcohol tolerance.

Metabolic tolerance occurs when the body can rapidly remove alcohol from its system. Enzymes in the the liver metabolize, or break down, the alcohol so it can exit the body. Metabolic tolerance is often seen in **chronic** drinkers. Their bodies remove alcohol faster, meaning the effects of the alcohol do not last as long. Tolerance of this type involves molecular and cellular adaptations that occur when a person starts drinking. They continue to adapt as more alcohol enters the body.

The second type of tolerance is **functional tolerance.** This refers to a person's ability to properly function when alcohol is present. The body, and in particular the brain, finds a way to work properly even when alcohol is in the system. As a result, larger quantities of alcohol

How Tolerance Can Be Learned

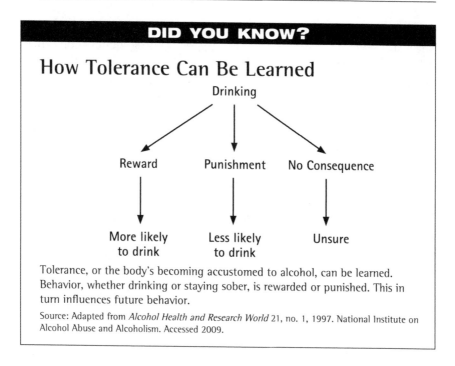

Drinking

Reward   Punishment   No Consequence

More likely   Less likely   Unsure
to drink   to drink

Tolerance, or the body's becoming accustomed to alcohol, can be learned. Behavior, whether drinking or staying sober, is rewarded or punished. This in turn influences future behavior.

Source: Adapted from *Alcohol Health and Research World* 21, no. 1, 1997. National Institute on Alcohol Abuse and Alcoholism. Accessed 2009.

are needed before a person becomes impaired. Usually, it takes time for functional tolerance to develop.

Acute tolerance occurs during a drinking session. At the beginning of the session, a person may be more impaired than later on. A person's blood alcohol content may be the same, but the body has rapidly adjusted to it and begins to function better.

The fourth type of tolerance is **learned tolerance**. Also referred to as "behaviorally augmented tolerance," learned tolerance is a process in which people acquire tolerance in less time. By practicing various tasks such as hand-eye coordination behaviors while under the influence of alcohol, the brain learns to overcome the impairments from alcohol.

The last two types of tolerance identified by the NIAAA are **environment-dependent tolerance** and **environment-independent tolerance**. Environment-dependent tolerance refers to someone developing and having alcohol tolerance in a particular setting. For example, someone who always drinks in a bar may have a higher tolerance for alcohol in that setting. However, in other settings, such as the home or a restaurant, the person's tolerance for alcohol is lower. By contrast, environment-independent tolerance refers to a person's tolerance of alcohol in any setting.

FACTORS INVOLVED IN ALCOHOL TOLERANCE

There are several factors that go into understanding alcohol tolerance. When alcohol is ingested, it binds to water molecules in the body. The amount of water in the body is partially dependent on a person's weight. Those who weigh more can absorb more alcohol before becoming impaired. However, those who have a higher percentage of body fat will have a lower tolerance because the alcohol cannot bind to the fat.

Research shows that other factors can influence one's tolerance of alcohol. For example, other drugs that can interfere with the effects of alcohol can increase a person's tolerance. A 2003 study in *Experimental and Clinical Psychopharmacology* reported on the effect caffeine has on alcohol tolerance. The authors found that when caffeine was given at the same time as alcohol, people performed at higher levels than those who were only given alcohol. Caffeine is a stimulant, whereas alcohol is a depressant. The presence of caffeine helped reduce, but not eliminate, the effects of alcohol on the brain.

A 2005 study in the journal *Experimental and Clinical Pharmacology* found that caffeine can help regulate behavior in someone who has been drinking. The authors found that people who were given alcohol alone had more difficulty completing tasks compared to people who were given alcohol and caffeine. In other words, caffeine can help block some of the effects of alcohol. However, the authors took this study a step further. They also compared both groups to a third group that was given alcohol and then given a monetary reward for properly completing tasks. This group also did better than the group receiving just alcohol. However, there were no significant differences between this group and the group given caffeine. In other words, given an incentive, such as money, to complete tasks while drinking was just as effective as consuming caffeine while drinking. This shows that, to some extent, tolerance can be learned.

The authors of a 2007 study in *Addiction Biology* explored the idea of tolerance following a history of alcohol dependence. The authors used rats in experiments to see if they still had a tolerance to alcohol following a period of abstinence from alcohol. There were two important findings. First, functional tolerance was still present. Second, however, metabolic tolerance was no longer present. In other words, soon after alcohol intake is stopped, the body's ability to break it down and remove it quickly from the system, disappears.

Q & A

Question: How do doctors learn about alcohol tolerance?

Answer: A lot of research studies are conducted with laboratory mice. Our understanding of genetics and our use of technology have advanced to the point where mice can be "designed" for research purposes. This is especially important because 99 percent of human genes also exist in mice.

Like humans, mice also have a complex central nervous system, thereby allowing researchers to study the effect alcohol has on the body without endangering the lives of people. One example comes from a 2008 study published in the journal *Alcohol*. The authors conducted tests with rats to see if chronic intermittent alcohol exposure in adolescence produces tolerance in adulthood. They found that high doses of alcohol did in fact influence subsequent tolerance against the effects of alcohol. In other words, repeated heavy exposure to alcohol during adolescence leads to a higher tolerance for alcohol as an adult, which in turn leads to heavier drinking.

LOSING TOLERANCE FOR ALCOHOL

Reverse tolerance happens when lower levels of alcohol are needed to create a reaction. Essentially, the person is losing tolerance for alcohol. This typically happens when there is liver damage. The liver is the primary organ that metabolizes alcohol. When damaged, it takes longer to metabolize alcohol, meaning it is easier for concentrations of alcohol to build up in the bloodstream. Reverse tolerance is typically found in people with a long history of alcohol abuse.

TEENS SPEAK

Binge Drinking Killed My Neighbor

I never really believed that drinking a lot at a party could kill anyone until my mother showed me this article in the local newspaper:

> An autopsy has determined that an 18-year-old college student found dead at a banned upstate fraternity

house had a blood-alcohol content as high as 0.55 percent—nearly seven times the legal limit for driving. The autopsy on the young man included three blood alcohol readings ranging from 0.39 percent to 0.55 percent. Experts say a level of 0.40 percent would send a healthy person into a coma, while 0.50 percent would be lethal. Police say he drank heavily during a wild party at the house near the state college, where he was a freshman biology major.

That student was a kid named Ted who used to live down the street from me. I can't believe he's dead from drinking.

See also: Alcohol Abuse, The Risks of; Alcohol and Disease; Alcoholism, Causes of; Effects of Alcohol on the Body; Withdrawal, Effects of

FURTHER READING
Herten, Jeff. *An Uncommon Drunk: Revelations of a High Functioning Alcoholic.* Bloomington, Ind.: iUniverse. 2006.

■ TREATMENT
See: Recovery and Treatment; Self-Help Programs

■ UNDERAGE DRINKING

Underage drinking means the consumption of alcoholic beverages by anyone under 21. That is the minimum age in all 50 states to legally purchase alcohol, whether at retail stores, restaurants, or bars.

Some states have exceptions built into the law; for example, some married people under 21 may purchase alcohol. In 19 states, younger people may legally drink in certain limited circumstances, such as in their home with parents. In fact, parents are almost never prosecuted in any state for serving alcohol to their own children in their own home.

Some experts recommend lowering the drinking age to 18 or 19, especially in those states that raised it in the late 1980s. They note that the legal drinking age is lower in every other country in the world—16, 18, or 20 in most democratic countries. The ages in Canadian provinces vary between 18 and 19.

Dr. Ruth Engs, professor of Applied Health Sciences at Indiana University, is one of those who favors reducing the legal drinking age and teaching responsible drinking in schools. She claims that one of the reasons many young people drink irresponsibly is that "drinking is seen by these youth as an enticing 'forbidden fruit,' a 'badge of rebellion against authority,' and a symbol of adulthood." She points to the experiment of national **Prohibition** in the 1920s, which promoted widespread disrespect for law.

On the other side of the debate, those who support the current legal age point out that Prohibition did in fact reduce the total amount of drinking and alcohol abuse. They also claim that the age-18 drinking limit helps keep down the death toll from drunk driving car crashes. They say that the increase in the legal age to 21, which many states carried out the late 1980s, was the primary reason for a dramatic decline in teenage drunken driving crashes. That decline translates to 1,000 fewer teenage deaths per year. Putting the age back down to 18 or 19, they fear, would send the wrong signal to the nation's kids.

Whichever camp is right, both agree that the laws are not always strictly enforced. In a 2002 law enforcement campaign in Montgomery County, Maryland, 38 percent of underage decoys were able to purchase alcohol. Other states have reported similar findings.

WHO ARE THE YOUNG DRINKERS?

Despite the law, underage drinking is widespread. At every age level, across regional, gender, and ethnic lines, there are at least some kids who engage in casual drinking or occasional binges, and some who are alcoholics. By the time kids reach the 18 to 20 age group, alcohol behavior does not differ much from that of adults.

The National Survey on Drug Use and Health provides an interesting profile of underage drinkers. An estimated 10.7 million people between the ages of 12 and 20 drank alcohol in 2007. More than 7 million engaged in binge drinking, while 2.3 million were heavy drinkers.

Whites were most likely to drink, with 32 percent admitting to using alcohol in the past month. American Indians or Alaska Natives were second (28.3 percent), followed by those of multiple races (26.2 percent), then Hispanics (24.7 percent), then blacks (18.3 percent), and finally Asians (16.8 percent). Whites were also most likely to engage in binge drinking, with 22.4 percent admitting to binge drinking in the past month. In this case, blacks were least likely to report binge drinking, with only 8.4 percent acknowledging the behavior.

As with older groups, males between 12 and 20 were more likely to drink than females. Current alcohol use was similar, with 28.4 percent of males and 27.3 percent of females drinking in the past month. The biggest difference was for binge drinking, with 21.1 percent of males and 16.1 percent of females binge drinking during the past month.

Those at the older end of this age group were more likely to drink than those at the younger end. Almost 51 percent of those between 18 and 20 drank alcohol within the past 30 days. This compares to only 3.5 percent of children ages 12 and 13.

THE RISKS OF RAPID PROGRESSION

When people ask what you hope to be when you grow up, no one will answer "an alcoholic." But every year, teenagers who thought they could handle a few drinks fall into the trap.

Every year, about 230,000 teenagers enroll in treatment programs for alcohol abuse. Unfortunately, experts believe that for every kid who signs up, several others need treatment and don't get it. Nationwide, the National Institute for Alcohol Abuse and Alcoholism estimates that between 5.2 and 5.5 million teenager abuse alcohol.

Most of the kids entering treatment do not show the severe physical effects that long-term adult alcoholics do, but they are definitely addicted. The therapists who screen kids for addiction depend a lot on behavioral signs, such as how often the patient gets drunk, or how he or she manages relationships with others.

Researchers have found that the younger kids are when they start to drink, the greater their risk for rapid progression to alcohol **abuse** and addiction. In other words, it takes younger kids less time to get addicted than older kids or adults. In 2003, the *American Journal of Psychiatry* published a review of many recent studies showing that adolescents may be more prone to alcohol and drug addiction, since their brains change more rapidly in response to a new stimulus (such as alcohol).

When kids drink heavily, even if they avoid actual addiction, they may be damaging their brain, according to other recent research. A 2002 article in the *Journal of Studies on Alcohol* reported that alcohol may interfere with brain development in adolescents, resulting in mild mental impairment. Alcohol-induced changes in the structure or size of the hippocampus (a key part of the brain) may cause lifelong memory problems.

Kids who start drinking young are more likely to have alcohol and other adjustment problems throughout their lives. In 2003 RAND

Health, an independent research institute, reported the results of a ten-year study; people who begin to drink by the seventh grade tend to show "employment problems, other substance abuse, and criminal and violent behavior" by age 23.

Of course, some of these people may have underlying problems that led to early drinking *and* later problems. Still, findings like these should make young people sit up and take notice.

WHAT HAPPENS AT 21?

The peak drinking age for Americans is 21. More people drink (71.8 percent in 2001), binge (50.1 percent), and are heavy drinkers (17.9 percent) at age 21 than at any point before or after, according to the 2007 National Household Survey on Drug Abuse. Young people who actually obeyed the laws, and delayed drinking until age 21, may be contributing to these high numbers.

A SERIOUS PROBLEM

More than half of all Americans have their first taste of alcohol before the legal purchasing age of 21. Unfortunately, too many of these underage drinkers have serious drinking problems. It is no exaggeration to say that underage alcohol abusers may be putting their futures at risk.

See also: Alcohol Poisoning; Effects on the Body; Law and Drinking, The; Peer Pressure and Alcohol

FURTHER READING

Merino, Noel. *Underage Drinking*. Chicago: Greenhaven Press, 2007.

Stewart, Gail B. *Teen Alcoholics*. San Diego, Calif.: Lucent, 2000.

Volkmann, Chris, and Toren Volkmann. *From Binge to Blackout: A Mother and Son Struggle with Teen Drinking*. New York: New American Library, 2006.

Windle, Michael. *Alcohol Use Among Adolescents*. Thousand Oaks, Calif.: Sage, 1999.

■ VIOLENCE AND ALCOHOL
See: Alcohol and Violence

■ WITHDRAWAL, EFFECTS OF

Body's often painful response to a decrease or stop in alcohol consumption. When someone drinks heavily over time, the body adjusts to the presence of alcohol, building up a tolerance. If a person significantly decreases, or stops, drinking alcohol, then the body goes into a state of shock. It must adjust once again, this time to the lack of alcohol. This readjustment period is formally known as alcohol withdrawal syndrome.

ALCOHOL WITHDRAWAL SYNDROME

The criteria for alcohol withdrawal syndrome are presented in the *DSM-IV,* the *Diagnostic and Statistical Manual of Mental Disorders, Fourth Edition,* published by the American Psychiatric Association. According to the *DSM-IV,* a person experiences alcohol withdrawal syndrome when at least two of the following conditions are met:

1. Autonomic hyperactivity (e.g., sweating, elevated pulse)
2. Increased hand tremor
3. Nausea or vomiting
4. Anxiety
5. Psychomotor agitation
6. Transient visual, tactile, or auditory hallucinations or illusion
7. Insomnia
8. Grand mal seizures

The autonomic nervous system (ANS) helps manage the body's response to stress. Autonomic hyperactivity means the ANS is working too hard. This causes an increase in blood pressure, an elevated breathing and heart rate, higher pulse, and an increase in body temperature, namely fever. Sweating can become so severe that a person has to worry about **dehydration.**

Alcohol withdrawal syndrome usually occurs within 24 to 48 hours, beginning within hours of stopping or reducing alcohol intake. Once again, it is important to state that withdrawal occurs after someone has engaged in prolonged and heavy drinking. Tremors occur between five to 10 hours after someone has had his or her last drink. Tremors typically reach their peak between 24 and 48 hours.

Chronic, or prolonged, drinking decreases the ability of the neurotransmitter GABA, in particular the GABAa neurotransmitter, to do its job. GABA plays an important role in sleep and maintaining lower levels of anxiety. It promotes a calm state and helps produce endorphins, which also provide a sense of well-being. GABA inhibits neurons in the brain from firing, or activating. Reducing brain activity helps promote calmness and well-being. Because GABA's ability to work properly has been compromised as a result of chronic alcohol exposure, the body has compensated accordingly. When the body starts withdrawing from the alcohol, the GABA neurotransmitters are still compromised and cannot help control anxiety, agitation, and nervousness.

The authors of a 2008 study in the *Journal of Neurology, Neurosurgery & Psychiatry* estimate that up to 86 percent of patients admitted to a hospital or other treatment facility for alcohol detoxification and rehabilitation will suffer from alcohol withdrawal. By the time someone has been admitted for alcohol abuse, he or she is likely to have been abusing alcohol for an extended period of time.

Typically, alcohol withdrawal occurs in people who have been abusing alcohol for at least three months. Those who drink excessive amounts of alcohol in a one-week period can also experience withdrawal.

Up to 25 percent of people withdrawing can experience "alcohol hallucinosis." The hallucinations can be visual, auditory (hearing), and tactile (feeling) in nature.

Those withdrawing can also experience "rum fits." These are the seizures that can occur during the withdrawal period. Up to 33 percent of patients experiencing withdrawal can have these rum fits. These seizures can progress to **delirium tremens** (DT's), terrifying hallucinations, for up to 5 percent of patients. DT's typically occurs 24 to 72 hours after a person has stopped drinking.

The authors of a 2008 article found on eMedicine note that there are approximately 1.2 million hospitalizations per year for problems related to alcohol abuse, including alcohol withdrawal syndrome. Of these, up to 5 percent may develop delirium tremens.

Delirium tremens is a severe symptom, if not the most severe symptom, of withdrawal. Some have referred to it as "the horrors" or "the fears." According to Medline Plus, an online resource provided by the National Institutes of Health and the U.S. National Library of Medicine, delirium tremens involves sudden and severe mental or neurological changes. If withdrawal has progressed to this point, the top goal of treatment is to save the person's life.

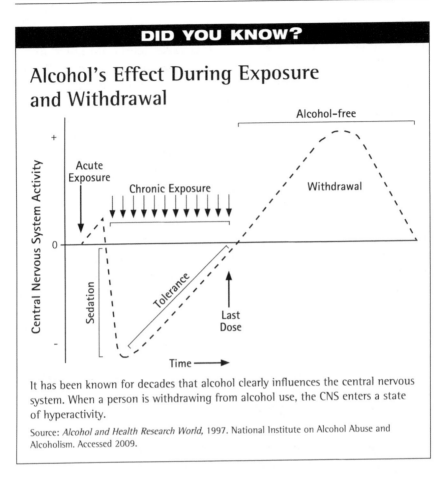

DID YOU KNOW?

Alcohol's Effect During Exposure and Withdrawal

It has been known for decades that alcohol clearly influences the central nervous system. When a person is withdrawing from alcohol use, the CNS enters a state of hyperactivity.

Source: *Alcohol and Health Research World,* 1997. National Institute on Alcohol Abuse and Alcoholism. Accessed 2009.

Delirium tremens in patients can lead to a heart attack because of an imbalance in the body's electrolytes. Patients have to be hooked up to cardiac monitors, given oxygen, and receive intravenous medications. Patients may also be sedated for up to a week while the body goes through the withdrawal process.

It is also important to know about the kindling phenomenon and alcohol withdrawal. Long-term changes in neurons found in the brain result from repeated detoxing. This results in an increase in alcohol craving and obsessive thoughts. This is why it becomes more difficult to withdraw from alcohol if that has been done before.

A 2007 article in the journal *Medical Science Monitor* adds some insight into the kindling phenomenon. The authors found that alcohol cravings during the withdrawal process are related to kindling. It is important to address cravings during the withdrawal process in order to minimize the chances of drinking after withdrawal.

Fact Or Fiction?

Can a person die from alcohol withdrawal?

The Facts: Yes, according to a 2008 report in *The Foundation Years*, more than 15 percent of people suffering from alcohol withdrawal used to die in the past. Due to better treatments, however, that number has dropped to 2 percent. Still, 8 percent of people die if they develop DT's.

TREATING ALCOHOL WITHDRAWAL SYNDROME

There are medications that can be used to treat people suffering from alcohol withdrawal syndrome. One class of drugs, **benzodiazepines,** has been shown to help because this class of drugs acts as a sedative. Studies have indicated these medications help with the overall symptoms of AWS and reduce the chances of seizures and delirium from occurring.

Barbiturates, such as phenobarbital, also work well. They can be used when the benzodiazepines are not working. Barbiturates have a longer-lasting effect.

Another drug that is useful for AWS is **carbamazepine.** This is an anti-seizure medication that has successfully been used in Europe for a some time and helps patients with mild to moderate levels of AWS.

Usually patients with AWS receive **thiamine,** also known as vitamin B1. Thiamine is depleted during alcohol use. This vitamin helps prevent patients from developing two conditions known as **Wernicke's encephalopathy** and **Korsakoff's psychosis.**

Wernicke's encephalopathy is a condition characterized by confusion, **ophthalmoplegia** (paralysis or weakness in at least one of the eye muscles), and **ataxia** (lack of coordination). Korsakoff's psychosis can damage the neurons in the brain, which may become a lifelong condition. The psychosis is characterized by anterograde and retrograde amnesia, invented memories (known as confabulation), lack of insight, apathy, and meager content in conversation. According to a 2008 article in the *Journal of Neurology, Neurosurgery & Psychiatry,* if doctors fail to identify Wernicke's encephalopathy and thiamine deficiency in their patients, there is a 20 percent mortality rate. The symptoms of AWS, therefore, can be extremely dangerous. It is best

DID YOU KNOW?

The Kindling Process

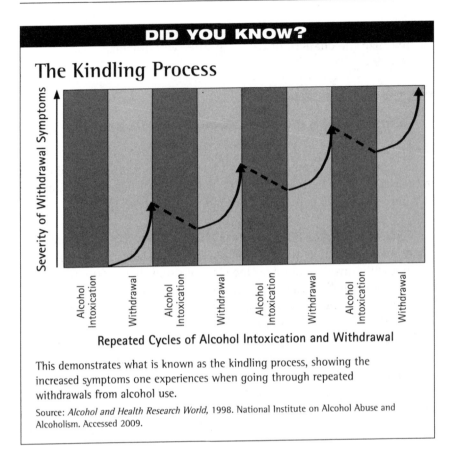

Severity of Withdrawal Symptoms

Alcohol Intoxication | Withdrawal | Alcohol Intoxication | Withdrawal | Alcohol Intoxication | Withdrawal | Alcohol Intoxication | Withdrawal

Repeated Cycles of Alcohol Intoxication and Withdrawal

This demonstrates what is known as the kindling process, showing the increased symptoms one experiences when going through repeated withdrawals from alcohol use.

Source: *Alcohol and Health Research World,* 1998. National Institute on Alcohol Abuse and Alcoholism. Accessed 2009.

to enter a hospital or special center for treatment, and it is important for nurses and doctors to closely monitor their patients.

See also: Alcoholism, Causes of; Effects of Alcohol on the Body; Recovery and Treatment; Tolerance and Reverse Tolerance

FURTHER READING

Klopocka, Maria, Jacek Budzynski, Maciej Swiatkowski, Grzegorz Pulkowski, and Marcin Ziolkowski. *Systematic and Metabolic Changes Observed in Alcohol Dependent Male Patients After Alcohol Withdrawal.* Hauppauge, N.Y.: Nova Science Publishers. 2009.

HOTLINES AND HELP SITES

Alateen
URL: http://www.al-anon.alateen.org/alateen.html
Phone: 1-888-4AL-ANON (8 A.M.–6 P.M. EST, M–F) or check the Web site for contact information in your area
Affiliation: part of Al-Anon, an organization of relatives and friends of alcoholics
Program: regular meetings of young people to discuss their problems and help each other face them
Mission: to help young people deal with problems of alcoholism in their families or among friends. Members meet in small local groups to discuss their problems and provide mutual support

Alcoholics Anonymous
URL: http://www.aa.org
Phone: 1-877-934-2522
Program: Worldwide fellowship of men and women from all walks of life who meet together to attain and maintain sobriety.
Mission: To stay sober and help other alcoholics achieve sobriety.

Alcohol Treatment Referral Hotline
Phone: 1-800-ALCOHOL (24 hours a day, 7 days a week)

American Council on Alcoholism
URL: http://www.aca-usa.org/
Phone: 1-800-527-5344 (Alcoholism Treatment HelpLine)

Center for Substance Abuse Treatment
URL: http://findtreatment.samhsa.gov/facilitylocatordoc.htm (helps locate the appropriate treatment facilities in your area)
Phone: 1-800-662-HELP (Referral Helpline, 24 hours a day, 7 days a week)
Affiliation: U.S. Department of Health and Human Services
Mission: to develop and promote better treatment for substance abuse

Freevibe
URL: http://freevibe.com/
Affiliation: National Youth Anti-Drug Media Campaign
Mission: to provide information to young people about alcohol and drugs, and to help kids find alternative interests and activities—"anti-drugs"

MADD Youth in Action
URL: http://www.madd.org/madd_programs/0,1056,2044,00.html
Affiliation: Mothers Against Drunk Driving (MADD)
Programs: Students around the country work with adults, with law enforcement officers, or with other students to prevent drunk driving.

National Association for Children of Alcoholics (NACoA) Just for Kids
URL: http://www.nacoa.org/kidspage.htm
Mission: aims to help kids whose parents abuse alcohol

National Council on Alcoholism and Drug Dependence (NCADD)
URL: http://www.ncadd.org/facts/youdir.html
Phone: 1-800-622-2255 (24-hour "hope line" for referral to local groups that can help); or 1-800-654-HOPE (National Intervention Network, to help people who need but do not want help with alcohol problems)
Affiliation: independent nonprofit group founded by alcoholics
Mission: supplies information about all aspects of alcohol and drugs; runs advocacy programs in New York and Washington to help alcoholics and drug addicts and fight addiction

Pages for Kids
URL: http://www.nacoa.org/kidspage.htm
Affiliation: U.S. Department of Health and Human Services

Mission: provide information to kids on all health-related issues; interactive activities and features

Students Examining the Culture of College Drinking
URL: http://findtreatment.samhsa.gov/facilitylocatordoc.htm
Affiliation: National Institute of Alcoholism and Alcohol Abuse
Mission: providing information about alcohol use and abuse for college students; helpful information for all teens, including interactive and multimedia features and additional help sites

GLOSSARY

A.A., or Alcoholics Anonymous   the world's first and largest self-help group for alcoholics

abstinence   the practice of not drinking any alcoholic beverages

abuse   to misuse a substance or to mistreat or cause injury to a person

acetaldehyde   a fairly toxic chemical produced by the liver when alcohol is **metabolized;** it can cause numerous unpleasant side effects

acetaminophen   a pain-relief and anti-inflammatory drug sold under various brand names such as Tylenol; it can harm the liver if taken together with or right after alcohol

acute tolerance   rapid adjustment during a drinking session to alcohol in the body; after initial impairment, the drinker begins to function better

adipose tissue   body fat; even moderate drinking can cause a buildup of fat if added to a normal diet

addiction   a condition in which a person habitually gives in to a psychological or physical need for a substance such as alcohol, tobacco, or drugs

AIDS   acquired immunodeficiency disease; an illness that destroys a person's immune system if left untreated; it is usually transmitted sexually

alcohol expectancy   a theory to explain the association of alcohol with violence or sex; people who believe that alcohol all by itself can turn a drinker violent or increase his or her sexual desire may become violent or sexually aggressive when they drink

alcohol psychosis   a bout of severe mental illness caused by long-term heavy drinking, often experienced during **withdrawal** and characterized by delusions, violence, convulsions, and other symptoms

alcoholic, alcoholics   a person who has a physical and psychological dependence on alcohol

amphetamines   a class of mood-changing drugs often used illegally; taken together with alcohol, they can cause severe stomach distress; by keeping drinkers awake, they can lead to dangerous overdoses of alcohol

anorexia nervosa   a medical/psychological condition in which the patient is unwilling to eat the minimum amount of food necessary to stay alive and healthy due to the mistaken idea that they are obese; sometimes associated with abuse of alcohol

Antabuse   an **aversion drug** widely used to treat alcoholics

antagonist   any drug that prevents alcohol from giving the drinker a high

aphrodisiac   any food or drink said to increase love or sexual desire

ataxia   lack of coordination

aversion drugs   any drug that makes people ill when they drink alcohol, used in treating **alcoholism**

BAC, or blood alcohol concentration   the percentage of alcohol in a fixed volume of blood

BAL, or blood alcohol level the percentage of alcohol in a fixed volume of blood

barbiturate(s) drugs used to treat seizures and delirium associated with alcohol withdrawal syndrome

benzodiazepine(s) drugs used to treat seizures and delirium associated with alcohol withdrawal syndrome

bipolar disorder a brain disorder that causes extreme shifts in a person's energy, mood, and ability to function; also known as manic-depressive illness

bootleggers smugglers and wholesale sellers of illegal alcohol during **Prohibition**

bulimia a medical/psychological condition in which the patient subjects his or her body to cycles of binge eating followed by vomiting or other extreme measures to get rid of the excess food; often associated with **alcohol abuse**

carbamazepine anti-seizure medication that is useful for patients with mild to moderate levels of alcohol withdrawal syndrome, or AWS

chronic long-lasting or repeated, used to describe any illness such as **alcoholism** that is not easily cured

chugging drinking a large quantity of alcohol in as short a time as possible; in other words, drinking faster than the body can process alcohol safely

congeners organic chemicals found in small amounts in alcoholic beverages; they can add flavor, but they also make a hangover worse

conditioning any routine, repeated experience that shapes a person's behavior; for example, people who grow up with parents who drink heavily may be conditioned to consider such behavior normal

counterconditioning any **behavioral therapy** that attempts to **condition** someone to change a behavior that the patient was previously conditioned to adopt

cross-addiction addiction to one drug as a substitute when another drug is unavailable; heroin addicts may be cross-addicted to alcohol

cross-tolerance a tolerance to one drug that makes the user tolerant to other drugs as well, even those he or she has never used

cure a complete recovery from a medical or psychological disease without any risk of its return

date rape forced sexual activity during a voluntary date

delirium tremens (the D.T.'s) intense, terrifying hallucinations that can accompany **withdrawal,** accompanied by high fevers and extremely aggressive behavior

dependence, dependency an intense physical or psychological need for a substance, such as alcohol; without the substance, a dependent person suffers severe discomfort or illness

depressant a drug that lowers the level of mental and physical activity

detoxification a course of treatment, usually at a hospital or other facility, aimed at freeing people from alcohol or drug abuse and restoring their bodies to good health

disease theory the idea that **alcoholism** is a disease rather than a moral failing or a lifestyle choice

disinhibition model a theory to explain the association of alcohol with violence; alcohol chemically blurs or deadens the parts of the brain that inhibit, or hold back, one's first impulsive reactions

distill to refine a beverage by heating it and directing the steam into another container where it is condensed back into liquid form

domestic abuse the repeated mistreatment of a family member or loved one; can be physical, emotional, or sexual

drug interactions   the combined effect on the body that two or more drugs have when used at the same time, for example, alcohol and various prescription drugs

dysfunctional   abnormal or unhealthy interpersonal behavior or interaction

enabling behaviors   actions whereby family, friends, and associates of a chemically dependent individual allow that individual, or enable him or her, to continue the addiction to alcohol or drugs

environment-dependent tolerance   the inability of a person to handle alcohol in a certain setting

environment-independent tolerance   the ability of a person to handle alcohol regardless of the place in which he or she is drinking

ethanol   the chemical name for drinking alcohol

false positive   a test result in which a person is found to have a problem with alcohol or drugs, even though one does not exist

false negative   a test result in which a person is found not to have a problem with alcohol or other substances when one does exist

fermentation   the natural chemical process in which nonalcoholic liquids such as fruit juice or grain mash are turned into alcoholic beverages; the sugar in the mixture turns to alcohol in the presence of yeast

fetal alcohol syndrome (FAS)   a group of birth abnormalities caused by drinking during pregnancy; it can include physical deformities and behavioral problems

functional tolerance   a state in which the body, and in particular the brain, finds a way to work properly even when alcohol is in a person's system

GABA   a neurotransmitter in the brain that plays an important role in sleep and maintaining low levels of anxiety; its effectiveness is interrupted by alcohol

gateway drug the first drug, often alcohol, used by people who later use illegal drugs

hallucination a sight or sound of something that is not really there

hazing physical or emotional abuse as part of an initiation process for new members of a college fraternity or other group

histamine one of the most important **congeners** found in alcoholic beverages

HIV human immunodeficiency virus, the organism that causes AIDS

hops a plant added in the brewing process to add flavor, color, and aroma to beer

illicit drugs drugs that are not legal for consumption, or that are used without a prescription for nonmedical reasons

intoxication impaired judgment caused by excessive alcohol consumption

kindling the progressive worsening of symptoms each additional time an alcoholic goes through withdrawal

learned tolerance process in which people acquire rapid tolerance of alcohol; by practicing various tasks such as hand-eye coordination behaviors while under the influence of alcohol, the brain learns to overcome the impairments from alcohol

malting the first stage in the process of brewing beer, in which grain kernels are allowed to sprout

marker a warning sign of a possible serious behavior problem; for example, drinking at a very young age is considered a marker for illegal drug use later

metabolic tolerance a natural process in which the liver learns to break down, or **metabolize,** a larger amount of a substance, such as alcohol, in a given period of time

metabolism, or metabolize   the process of breaking down a substance in the body, or to break down a substance in the body

methanol   a common **congener** in alcoholic beverages; some believe it is the main cause of a hangover

morality theory   the idea that people become alcoholics through weak morals; it was popular in the 18th and 19th centuries

Mothers Against Drunk Driving (MADD)   an advocacy group that tries to reduce drunk driving by stronger laws and law enforcement and by information campaigns

Naltrexone   a drug widely used to treat alcoholics

nicotine   the addictive substance found in tobacco

ophthalmoplegia   paralysis or weakness in at least one of the eye muscles

platelet   a type of blood cell that helps heal wounds; heavy drinking may reduce a person's platelet level

progression   movement from one stage of **alcohol dependency** to a more intense, dangerous stage

progressive illness   a condition, such as **alcohol abuse,** that tends to get worse with time

Prohibition   in the United States from 1919 to 1933, the complete ban on the sale or drinking of alcohol

proof   the proportion of alcohol in a given beverage; figured as twice the percentage by volume: a 100 proof beverage is 50 percent alcohol by volume; used in the United States

psychosis   a mental disorder that includes hallucinations and delusions

psychotherapy   a course of treatment, often based on discussion between a patient and a doctor or counselor, aimed at helping patients modify their behaviors and/or improve their mental states

rape sex without consent, usually by force

recovering alcoholic according to the disease model of alcoholism, any alcoholic who is currently abstaining or trying to abstain from alcohol

recreational drug a drug used to get high or change one's mood

resveratrol a chemical found in red wine that may help prevent aging in moderate drinkers

risk factor anything, such as family background or personal problems, that might put a person at high risk for alcohol abuse or other dangerous outcome

sexually transmitted disease (STD) any disease that can be passed from one person to another during sexual relations

sobriety abstaining from alcohol (or other addictive drug)

social drinking moderate drinking in a social context

speakeasy illegal bar in the **Prohibition** era

stepping-stone a drug whose users will often move on to another, more dangerous drug, according to some researchers; for example, alcohol is considered by some to be a stepping-stone to marijuana

stimulant a drug that makes you feel wide-awake and full of energy

substance abuse any unhealthy or unsafe use of alcohol, illegal drugs, prescription drugs, or any other chemical

syndrome any collection of unhealthy symptoms or behaviors that usually appear together

tagging the practice of marking beer kegs by the seller so that kegs found at parties of underage students can be traced back to the source

temperance movement a movement that arose in England and the United States in the 18th century to advocate moderation in drinking;

eventually, some temperance supporters became advocates of **prohibition**

thiamine also known as vitamin B1, it is depleted in the brain as a result of frequent and heavy alcohol use, leading to neurological disorders and psychosis

tolerance the state in which the body has become accustomed to alcohol or another substance, so that a person needs to drink more to get the same mental effect

toxic poisonous

tremors shaking

twelve-step program any treatment program for alcoholism or other addiction that stresses the Twelve Steps to recovery developed by A.A. (Alcoholics Anonymous)

tyramine a chemical found naturally in beer and red wine, that can dangerously increase blood pressure if a drinker also uses MAOI antidepressants

venereal disease former term for **sexually transmitted disease**

Volstead Act the 1919 law that put **Prohibition** into effect in the United States

Wernicke's encephalopathy a condition characterized by confusion, **ophthalmoplegia** (paralysis or weakness in at least one of the eye muscles), and **ataxia** (lack of coordination)

zero tolerance a policy of enforcing and prosecuting even the most minor incidence of any law, such as drunk-driving or drug-possession laws

INDEX

Boldface page numbers indicate extensive treatment of a topic.